The Opiate Cure

The Opiate Cure

Pain and the Bipolar Spectrum

Robert T. Cochran Jr., MD

To order additional copies of this book, contact:
Xlibris Corporation
1-888-795-4274
www.Xlibris.com
Orders@Xlibris.com
102652

CONTENTS

To those who suffer from chronic pain and bipolar disorder
and the stigma of taking a drug that cures

PREFACE

About four years ago, I had both knees replaced. The operation and my convalescence were uncomplicated except for an issue that distressed me greatly. I couldn't sleep. Each night, my mind was overwhelmed with memories of pleasurable experiences—biking, skiing, backpacking, and fishing with friends and family. I quickly grew tired of remembering the happy times. I wanted desperately to be able to sleep, but I could not. My mind was too busy, and for the only time in my life, a force beyond my control was commanding my thoughts. Only after several days at home was I able to think as I wished as I awaited sleep. What had happened to me? I want to suggest to you that I experienced just a touch of bipolar mania. The appearance of mania after a surgical operation is by no means unheard of. And characteristics of mania are sleeplessness, mind busyness, and sometimes obsessive and repetitive thought. Bipolar mania makes us think what we don't want to think, and that is what happened to me. I do not, by any conventional standard of measure, suffer from bipolar disorder; but I want to suggest to you that maybe all of us, at some time or another in our lives, become a little bit bipolar, especially when we are in pain. Keep that in mind as you read this book.

I am indebted to many people for their assistance in preparing this work. Donna, my wife of many years, has once again given me time and space to write about something that I think is quite important. I have been supported greatly during the time of this writing by my office staff. Their names are Jan Diehl, Janet Epstein, Linda Harris, Pat Alley, Renee Turman, Tammy Gohlson, and B. J. Tucker. I have also been supported by my transcriptionist, Sherry Jolly, who does the important little things for me, like spelling and punctuating. I am indebted to the many physicians who have referred their difficult patients to me. As you will see in this book, my referrals come from across the spectrum of medical specialists—all the way from psychiatrists to urologists. Thus, it has been my privilege to see people with a remarkable variety of painful disorders. Lastly, I express my gratitude to my patients who have taught me so much. I hope this book will express my devotion and the respect I hold for them. It is their stories that I offer you in the certain knowledge that as you read of others, you will find yourself and will be comforted by the fact that you are not alone, that there is hope for recovery, and that you need not be ashamed of taking pain pills.

INTRODUCTION

For those of you unfamiliar with my writings on the subject of chronic pain, I will briefly summarize them and in doing so introduce you to this work.

In 2004, I published my first book, *Understanding Chronic Pain*. I accepted the generally held belief that chronic pain could best be defined as pain that extends beyond the anticipated time of recovery from illness or injury. I pointed out, however, that when this happens, there appears, almost invariably, a host of other symptoms in addition to the pain. These include disordered sleep, appetite, energy, mood, thought, memory, and even motor skills. I emphasized that these symptoms coexist so frequently with chronic pain that they must be considered inherent to the disease; and it matters not whether the painful state is fibromyalgia, headache, back pain, neuritis, arthritis, or whatever. Clearly, there is great commonality among those who suffer from chronic pain. For this reason and others, I suggested that although chronic pain may appear in a variety of forms, it represents a single core illness. I suggested also that the illness could be best considered a disorder of the mind. The reasons for this are several. Chronic pain is often preceded by the psychiatric disorders of substance abuse and depression and also very commonly by childhood trauma—particularly sexual abuse, which, as you may know, is the mother of many psychiatric diseases. Moreover, chronic pain often coexists with a psychiatric illness, including depression, panic, bipolar disorder, attention deficit disorder, post-traumatic stress disorder, obsessive-compulsive disorder, multiple personality disorder, and others. In my book, I presented the case histories of people with chronic pain who were successfully treated by the introduction of *psychopharmacy* (drugs for the mind). I concluded that recognition and treatment of the coexistent (*comorbid* is the medical term) psychiatric disease could often relieve pain.

My book did well, and 2006 found me working on a second edition. Mainly, I was pleased with my work. My ideas seemed to be standing the test of time, at least as measured over a couple of years. Therefore, I made no major revisions in the new edition. Nonetheless, a couple of lines of thought were evolving: one related to the role of opiate therapy and the other to bipolar disorder. Let's take bipolar first.

I had written about a man whose recurrent back pain went away when his bipolar disease was treated with Lithium. Thus, I did appreciate a link between the two diseases, but I thought the effect was probably quite rare because (I believed then) the incidence of bipolarity in the population at large was only about 2 or 3 percent. However, as time went by and I learned more about bipolar disorder, I began to recognize the very great frequency of bipolarity in my patients with chronic pain. Moreover, I found myself becoming more comfortable and confident in treating people who suffer from both pain and bipolarity. The reader is advised that that can be an intimidating combination. The victims of bipolar disorder are brittle emotionally, behaviorally, and also pharmacologically. Their responses to drug therapy are often adverse and unpredictable. Drugs that should make them better can make them worse. Moreover, there is a high incidence of drug abuse in the bipolar population. (Some 50 percent of heroin addicts are bipolar!)

It was in the summer of 2006 that I first learned of the emerging concept of the *bipolar spectrum*. Psychiatrists were recognizing that bipolar disorder was often linked—that is to say, comorbid—with narcolepsy, migraine, attention deficit disorder (ADD), and obsessive-compulsive disorder (OCD). There was also increasing awareness that bipolarity and chronic pain in their many forms were often comorbid. I bought into the concept quickly because it fit with so many of my own ideas, but I did strike out a couple of times. I should have appreciated a link between bipolarity and migraine because I was seeing plenty of both, but I didn't make the connection. In but a short while, however, I realized that migraine is quite common in the bipolar, and it is often severe and treatment resistant. The link to narcolepsy had escaped me entirely, but I did recall that some of my patients did complain of vivid threatening dreams, a hallmark of narcolepsy.

I was sure the concept of the bipolar spectrum was correct. I accepted unreservedly the *clinical* link—that is, the simultaneous existence of some or all of these disorders in one person. And I knew also that there was very likely a *genetic* link. Bipolarity is often a familial disease, and many of my bipolars in pain had children with ADD. Now could there be a *therapeutic* link? That is, could the treatment of one disorder in the spectrum relieve the others? Particularly, what would be the role of *psychostimulant* (Ritalin is an example) therapy? The psychostimulants are indicated in the treatment of both attention deficit disorder and narcolepsy. What would be their place in the treatment of bipolar disorder, chronic pain in general, and migraine in particular? I knew I would find out pretty soon.

My opportunity came when a woman with arthritic knee pain was referred to me. She was bipolar and had spent years on treatment with many drugs. She told me that as her pain had appeared and was progressively worsening, she had developed a problem with mood shifts (bipolarity), forgetfulness, want of mental focus, and distractibility (ADD). In response to my questioning, she reported that she had throughout her life been subject to vivid dreams. Moreover, she was fatigued and sleepy in the daytime (narcolepsy). I felt I had limited treatment choices. I certainly wasn't going to employ conventional psychopharmacy because she had already been on most of the drugs I use, and many of them had made her worse. That left opiates for her pain or stimulants for her attention deficiency and narcolepsy. Fearful (at that time) of opiates in the bipolar, I prescribed Ritalin knowing that it might precipitate mania. But I also knew that any drug I chose might precipitate mania. It wasn't a very attractive choice, but I thought it was the best. The only other option was to tell her I had nothing to offer, and I don't like doing that. Her recovery was sudden and total. Within but days, her pain was relieved, her distractibility diminished, her energy restored, her sleepiness overcome, and, in short order, her nightmares went away. Astonishingly also, her mood shifts were arrested.

Encouraged, to say the least, by her response, I continued to pursue the role of psychostimulant therapy. I encountered a young woman with accelerating migraine and also anxiety and, with them, the appearance of nightmares. Again, the improvement with stimulant therapy was dramatic. Her migraines disappeared, and her anxiety level was diminished. I was also to discover later that her dental phobia was totally abated. She could attend, under the sponsorship of my therapy with Ritalin, a dental appointment without fear or anxiety. Next I encountered a patient with migraine who also suffered from obsessive-compulsive disorder, which was only partially responsive to treatment. She reported very threatening dreams. I introduced stimulant therapy, and not only were her migraines and dreams diminished, but her obsessive-compulsive disorder also.

It had not taken long to validate, at least in my mind, the concept of the bipolar spectrum. It made bipolarity bigger and more complex than I had thought, but also more vulnerable. There were more points of attack.

Now back to opiates. In *Understanding Chronic Pain*, I had largely neglected, perhaps even disparaged, the use of opiates. I worried (probably too much) about addiction. A bigger issue was that the opiates, I thought then, were rather ineffective in the treatment of chronic pain. Such was my enthusiasm for the role of psychopharmacy that I wrote that the victim of chronic pain can actually get well or nearly so with those drugs. The victim of chronic pain did not get well with opiates, only a bit better until it was time for another pill. Nonetheless, one cannot be a pain doctor and not use opiates, and as time was going by, I was becoming more knowledgeable about the opiates and more aggressive in their use. Whereas formerly I had chosen to employ the weakest—and presumably least addictive—opiates, I had, with increasing experience, begun to employ stronger ones in bigger doses and often in combination. I finally realized that the generous prescription of opiates can reduce human suffering; and that, I concluded, should include *bipolar* human suffering.

A man who had endured multiple spinal operations and had chronic back pain was referred to me. He had become extremely obese, for chronic pain is often a food-craving, weight-gaining disease. With his pain, he had evolved, as is so often the case, into unstable bipolarity with depression, suicidal ideation, and periods of manic hyperactivity and anger requiring hospitalizations and, on one occasion, incarceration. He was under psychiatric care, receiving multiple drugs without much success. I was not attracted to giving him more, so I elected to simply prescribe morphine for his pain. Within days, his pain was relieved, and his mood was stabilized in a manner he had not known for years on conventional therapy. Moreover, his lust for sweets was abated, and he started losing weight rapidly.

Next a woman in her forties who had been raped and shot in the neck by her ex-husband. The carotid artery was damaged but surgically repaired without incident. The bullet, however, remained lodged in the vertebral column, and surgery to remove it would carry a high risk of paralysis. Her neck remained painful, and she required the use of a thick collar to prevent painful neck movement. Within a few months of her assault, she developed post-traumatic stress disorder with anxiety, depression, and terrifying flashbacks of the event. She attempted suicide and required hospital admission. While there, her mood-shifting bipolar disorder was recognized and treated. However, in spite of aggressive psychiatric care with many medications, she remained anxious, angry, painful, and mood unstable. I prescribed Morphine. On her return, she reported that she didn't hurt quite as badly, but that little else had changed. I probably should have increased the dose of Morphine. It was helping a bit, and she was having no significant side effects; but for reasons still uncertain to me, I elected to add another opiate, Methadone. On her return, she was unencumbered by the collar. She moved about gracefully, and she told me with a radiant smile that I had cured her. The pain was gone; and so were her anxiety, depression, and mood shifts. Moreover, she was no longer having flashbacks.

I had, within the course of but a month, seen two unstable bipolars whose disease was totally and suddenly arrested by the administration of opiates. Both of them were clinical miracles, and one does occasionally see a random clinical miracle. But two nearly identical miracles in one month are not random. I did some research and discovered that in the first half of the twentieth century, before the advent of our contemporary pharmacy for psychiatric disease, Morphine was sometimes used for the treatment of depression, mania, and delirium. Occasionally, it worked. The effect was called the *opiate cure*.

Once again the bipolar spectrum was validated. Just think about it. By employing a stimulant in persons with narcolepsy or attention deficiency and employing an opiate in persons with chronic pain, I had not only relieved the pain of arthritis, migraine, a multiply-operated low back, and a bullet in the neck, I had also cured or ameliorated bipolar disorder, obsessive-compulsive disorder, attention deficit disorder, phobia, post-traumatic stress disorder, narcolepsy, and even obesity! It beggars the imagination that all this could happen in only five patients. But it is true.

I knew I had to share these stories, and I began my second book, to be entitled *Curing Chronic Pain*. To a remarkable extent, I was learning as I was writing. So rapidly coming were new experiences and new ideas that at least a third of the material presented in the book, I did not know when I began writing it. Indeed, I found it difficult to end the book because almost daily, it seemed, there was a new experience and a new insight. Fortunately for me, the learning curve, which had been ascending at great velocity over the course of a couple of years, has slowed a bit; and that is good. It has given me time to gather my thoughts and process what I have learned. It has also given me time also to increase my database. My population of patients with chronic pain and the bipolar spectrum on treatment with opiates or stimulants (and sometimes both) has grown from a few dozen to several hundred. I have come to embrace the concept of the bipolar spectrum and, more importantly, its clinical application. By understanding the scope of the disease and its very common association with chronic pain, I am better able to treat both.

The acceptance of my ideas by those whom I have treated for chronic pain and bipolarity, usually quite successfully, has been enthusiastic. Others who have read my books or visited my Web site have also been accepting, and I will shortly share some of their e-mails with you. Among the medical community, however, acceptance has been much more hesitant. There are, I believe, many reasons for this—some good and some not so. One is the sheer improbability that stimulants, and especially opiates, can relieve such a host of different psychiatric disorders, even those that were resistant to conventional therapy, so quickly and so totally. It is too good to be true, and therefore, it challenges credulity. Moreover, if it is indeed true, why had we not recognized it sooner? The opiates have been around for millennia, stimulants for over a century. If their effects are as dramatic as I have written, why did we not see it? Actually, we had. The use of opiates for the treatment of mental illness was widely practiced throughout the Western world, perhaps most so in Germany, but certainly also in the United States. I will remind the reader that the only other treatment for severe mental illness in the opiate era was the *prefrontal lobotomy*, the surgical destruction of a portion of a person's brain. With the development of electroconvulsive therapy in the 1930s, and then effective psychopharmacy in the 1960s, both the opiate cure and the prefrontal lobotomy were consigned to oblivion. The prefrontal lobotomy fortunately so. The opiate cure—well, one wonders.

A bigger issue relating to the acceptance of opiate therapy for psychiatric disorders lies in our medical and societal attitudes toward the drugs. All agree that they are necessary for the relief of acute pain, and nearly all agree that they should also be employed in the long-term treatment of chronic pain. Nearly all also agree, the author and a few others excepted, that they have no other real clinical utility beyond the relief of pain. Moreover, they are dangerous to the person who uses them regularly because he will become addicted and to the doctor who prescribes them because he will lose his license. The extent of this fear cannot be overstated, and that is why so few doctors use opiates generously and therefore why so few doctors have the opportunity to witness the opiate cure.

I was for twenty years a pain doctor, prescribing opiates regularly, before I witnessed it. It was an exercise in *serendipity* (finding something good that you are not looking for). It was a chance discovery; but it was also, I believe, providential. It came at a time in my career when I had recognized the frequency of bipolarity in my patients in pain, when I had discovered the enormity of the bipolar spectrum, and when I was learning to administer opiates aggressively. The two unstable bipolars who experienced the opiate cure were not merely case studies. They were a *message* that there was a link between the bipolar spectrum, chronic pain, and perhaps uniquely to those disorders, opiate therapy. My patients got better *because* they were bipolar, and they probably also had pain *because* they were bipolar. Curious, and perhaps ironic, that the opiates—drugs that I had disparaged in print but four years before—were suddenly becoming my bedrock for the treatment of the bipolar in pain; and there are an awful lot of those out there.

CHAPTER 1

Drugs for Pain and the Bipolar Spectrum

I have elected, as in my previous books, to list in tabular form the drugs that will be referenced in this text. Many of my readers, most of whom have taken several of these drugs, tell me that this kind of overview at the beginning of the book is helpful.

Be advised that drugs of great variety are employed in the treatment of bipolarity and pain. Some of them have been approved by the Federal Drug Administration (FDA) for those purposes, but some have not. The latter usage derives from the not infrequent discovery that a new drug, indicated for the treatment of a specific symptom or disease, is often found to be effective in treating other symptoms and diseases. Thus, the prescription of drugs for non-FDA approved purposes, known as *off-label prescribing*, is widely recognized as appropriate and needful.

Most of the drugs discussed in this book influence the way nerve cells (neurons) within the brain communicate with each other. A chemical, the *neurotransmitter*, is released from one cell and attaches to a site, known as a *receptor*, on the surface of another cell. Virtually all of the brain's functions perform under the persuasion of neurotransmitters and their receptors. It is their dysfunction that is the cause of most neuropsychiatric illness; and it is correction of that dysfunction with pharmacy that allows us to relieve, or at least control, mental illness.

I discussed, at some length, neurotransmitters and their function in *Curing Chronic Pain*. I will not repeat that exercise, in part because I believe once is enough and in part also because this is really not my area of expertise. In this chapter, I will speak only briefly on the matter but will in text elaborate on it when it is appropriate.

Antidepressants

Selective Serotonin Reuptake Inhibitors (SSRI)

The SSRIs are the best known of the antidepressants. They enhance the activity of the nerve transmitter serotonin, which is the brain's own antidepressant. They also have antianxiety properties and have to a large measure supplanted the more conventional anxiolytics (tranquilizers) in the treatment of anxiety. Unfortunately, perhaps because of their selective serotonin activity, they are only modestly effective as analgesic (pain-relieving) drugs. They can be very effective in the bipolar although occasionally untoward reactions, particularly mania, can be generated by the SSRIs.

Proprietary	**Generic**
Celexa	Citalopram
Lexapro	Escitalopram
Luvox	Fluvoxamine
Paxil	Paroxetine
Prozac	Fluoxetine
Zoloft	Sertraline

Tricyclic and Tricyclic-like Antidepressants

These, the first widely used antidepressants clearly have pain-relieving attributes. This is because they increase not only the activity of serotonin but also noradrenaline, which is one of the brain's own pain-controlling nerve transmitters. They, perhaps more than any other class of drugs, carry the risk of the induction of mania in the bipolar. Nonetheless, they can be extremely helpful in victims of that disorder. More recently there have appeared tricyclic-like drugs, which are also effective for pain and bipolar depression. They are Effexor and Cymbalta. A kindred drug, known as Savella, has only recently been released. It appears to enhance only the activity of noradrenaline and has been FDA-approved for the treatment of the pain of fibromyalgia.

Proprietary	**Generic**
Anafranil	Clomipramine
Cymbalta	Duloxetine

Desipramine	Norpramine
Effexor	Venlafaxine
Elavil	Amitriptyline
Pamelor	Nortriptyline
Savella	Milnacipran
Sinequan	Doxepin
Tofranil	Imipramine

Dopamine Antidepressants

Dopamine, the brain's gratification, reward, and pleasure neurotransmitter is enhanced by dopamine antidepressants. A very similar effect is achieved by the psychostimulants, which will be addressed shortly.

Proprietary	**Generic**
Wellbutrin	Bupropion
Emsam	Selegiline

Anxiolytics

This group of drugs, also known as tranquilizers, belongs to a chemical class known as benzodiazepine. They enhance the activity of gamma-aminobutyric acid (GABA), which is the brain's calming and sedating neurotransmitter. Their use is disdained by many because of their potential for addiction. Nonetheless, they can be extremely helpful drugs in the treatment of pain. Those asterisked below particularly so, perhaps because of their anticonvulsant (antiepileptic) properties.

Proprietary	**Generic**
Ativan*	Lorazepam*
Klonopin*	Clonazepam*
Librium	Chlordiazepoxide
Restoril	Temazepam
Serax	Oxazepam
Tranxene	Clorazepate
Valium*	Diazepam*
Xanax	Alprazolam

Anticonvulsants

There are a great number of these drugs, and they all were released with the original indication for the treatment of epilepsy. All, virtually without exception, are useful also for the prevention of migraine and for the control of bipolar mood swings. They do not act on a specific neurotransmitter but, rather, render the nerve cell membrane, that which carries electrochemical message throughout the length of the cell, less volatile and irritable. It is this nerve cell irritability that is probably the root cause of epilepsy, migraine, mania, and perhaps also chronic pain, and the anticonvulsants are widely used for those disorders. Only one of the drugs listed below has no anticonvulsant activity, but it was historically the first drug (if we exclude the opiates) for the treatment of bipolar mania. It is Lithium.

Proprietary	Generic
Depakote	Valproate
Dilantin	Phenytoin
Keppra	Levetiracetam
Lamictal	Lamotrigine
Lithonate, Eskalith	Lithium
Lyrica	Pregabaline
Neurontin	Gabapentin
Tegretol	Carbamazepine
Topamax	Topiramate
Zonegran	Zonisamide

Antipsychotics

This group of drugs was originally designed for the treatment of schizophrenia. They also are useful for the treatment of agitation and delirium, particularly in the elderly with dementia. They appeared early on to have fewer of the troublesome side effects that accompanied the first antipsychotics (of which Thorazine, Prolixin, and Haldol will be referenced in this book). They were also discovered to be quite helpful in the treatment of bipolar disorder, and they are widely employed for that purpose. In recent years, however, there has come increasing awareness of the side effects of obesity and diabetes.

Proprietary	Generic
Abilify	Aripiprazole
Geodon	Ziprasidone
Risperdal	Risperidone
Seroquel	Quetiapine
Zyprexa	Olanzapine

Psychostimulants

These drugs, most derived from amphetamine, are widely used in the treatment of attention deficit disorder, narcolepsy, fatigue, daytime sleepiness, and occasionally, depression. They can be, as we have already seen, mood-stabilizing, anxiolytic, and migraine-preventing in the bipolar. Most of them enhance the activity of the neurotransmitter, dopamine (as does cocaine), and perhaps for this reason they carry the capacity for addiction. However, they also stimulate noradrenaline, and that may account for their occasional pain-relieving effects. Two of the psychostimulants are neither amphetamine-derived nor dopamine enhancers. Rather, they stimulate noradrenaline. They are widely used for the treatment of attention deficit disorder (Strattera) and excessive sleepiness (Provigil), but, curiously, their analgesic effect appears to be limited.

Proprietary	Generic
Adderall	Amphetamine
Adderall XR*	Amphetamine*
Dexedrine	Dextroamphetamine
Ritalin	Methylphenidate
Concerta*	Methylphenidate*
Focalin XR*	Dexmethylphenidate
Provigil	Modafinil
Strattera	Atomoxetine
Vyvanse	Lisdexamfetamine

*Extended Release Preparations

Antimigraine Drugs

These agents are collectively identified from a common chemical structure as triptan. They influence the activity of serotonin in blood vessels and not in the brain. They cause vascular constriction, and that opposes the pain-inducing vascular dilatation that is the hallmark of migraine. They will be referenced several times in this text.

Proprietary	Generic
Amerge	Naratriptan
Frova	Frovatriptan
Imitrex	Sumatriptan
Maxalt	Rizatriptan
Relpax	Eletriptan
Zomig	Zolmitriptan

Opioid Analgesics

Most of the pain-relieving opioids are derivative of the opium poppy (*papaver somniferum*) although some are prepared synthetically. They enhance the effect of the endorphins, the brain's own pain-relieving neurotransmitter. They are predictably effective in the treatment of the acute painful illness or injury but less so in those who suffer from chronic pain. The exception, as I will demonstrate throughout this book, is in those who suffer from pain and bipolar disorder. In that group of people, they can be not only pain-relieving, but also anxiety-diminishing, mood-stabilizing, depression-alleviating, attention-restoring, obsession-diminishing, and migraine-preventing. They are certainly the most addictive of the drugs referenced in this book, and their abuse is an enormous medical and societal problem. Nonetheless, I believe in the appropriate circumstance, and these are not few, their benefit can be remarkable. I am hopeful that the coming decades will witness the birth of the science of *opiate psychopharmacology*, the study of why and how opiates can be so helpful for mental illness, particularly for the bipolar spectrum and its many and varied expressions.

Two of the opiates, Buphrenorphine and Methadone, possess the capacity to inhibit withdrawal from heroin and other opiates and also to diminish cravings for those drugs. They are widely employed in the detoxification from opiates.

Proprietary	Generic
Darvon	Propoxyphene
Demerol	Meperidine

Dilaudid, Exalgo*	Hydromorphone
Duragesic,* Actiq, Fentora	Fentanyl
Lortab, Vicodin, Norco	Hydrocodone
Methadose	Methadone (Dolophine)
MS Contin,* Kadian,* Avinza,* MSIR	Morphine
Nubain	Nalbuphine
Opana, Opana ER*	Oxymorphone
Percodan, Tylox, Oxycontin*	Oxycodone
Stadol	Butorphanol
Suboxone	Buphrenorphine
Ultram	Tramadol

* Extended release preparation

Some of these drugs are formulated in combination with Tylenol, which is Acetaminophen. Their names are suffixed with—cet, thus, Lorcet, Percocet, Ultracet, and Darvocet, which has just, at the time of this writing, been withdrawn because of cardiac side effects.

I must, of necessity, address the frustrating and confusing issue of the duality of drug names, that is, generic or proprietary. My choices have been, I'll admit, inconsistent. I have elected to employ the generic name for the tricyclics and most of the opiates. They are old drugs, years removed from patent protection, and they are identified on the prescription label by their generic name. Other drugs, nearly as old, and I am referring to the SSRIs and the anxiolytics, are also identified on the prescription label by their generic names. Nonetheless, many have entered our cultural lexicon as branded products, and I am referring to Valium and Prozac. Therefore, I have chosen to employ brand names for those drugs and also the newer ones that are so identified on the prescription label. I believe this decision will make for easier reading because, by intent, brand names are shorter and easier to read, pronounce, and remember (think about Librium versus Chlordiazepoxide). I have elected to disobey the convention of placing proprietary names in the upper case and generic in the lower. I place all drug names in capitals just as I do in my medical records because it invites quick and easy attention.

Lastly, I must point out that in this book I will endorse, with great enthusiasm, the use of opiates for the treatment of the bipolar spectrum. This is about as non-FDA approved, off-label prescribing as one can get. That said, realize that I am prescribing opiates for the treatment of pain, and that is certainly FDA-approved. So what I present in this book is within FDA guidelines and is not off-label prescribing at all. If, in the process of prescribing FDA-approved drugs for the treatment of pain, I make providential and serendipitous discoveries, what is wrong with that?

CHAPTER 2

The Bipolar Way

An e-mail:

Dear Dr. Cochran:

My name is John Reynolds. I am 30 years old. I live in New Hampshire. I am bipolar, diagnosed at age 17. I have had migraines since I was 5 years old. About four years ago my headaches changed. They would come several times a day, and the pain was like nothing I have ever felt. It causes the right side of my face to turn red, and that side of my nose will plug up. The pain pinpoints in the corner of my eye and radiates around my entire eye into the cheekbone and jaw, and it feels like my teeth are being crushed. These come on frequently at night waking me up to one to four times. My dentist blamed the headache on my wisdom teeth, so I had them removed. I thought the pain was over, but a couple of months later the headache came back. I went back to the dentist, and he said the problem was in my jaw joint, and he gave me a guard to put in my mouth at night. That did no good at all. For a couple of years, my headaches would only occur occasionally. I would have them several times daily, most often at night, and they would come in clusters lasting two or three weeks at a time. Then I would have maybe a month or two with freedom from headaches.

That all changed a year and a half ago, and I now have what I am told is chronic cluster migraine. Eighteen months of up to eight headaches a day! They will last from five minutes to two or three hours. It is like I am being stabbed in my right eye. I will sometimes sit in the shower with washcloths on my face for a soothing effect. For a long while I was misdiagnosed as having chronic sinusitis. I was prescribed antibiotics that didn't work, and then my doctors began to give me drugs like Amitriptyline, but that made me manic. After several months with my doctor, I made the mistake of swearing at him on the answering machine during a headache and extreme pain. He discharged me after pointless, useless scripts and having me squirt saltwater up my nose four times daily for a year. Then I found a doctor who knew something about chronic cluster headaches. He gave me Imitrex, but that made me feel like I had glass in my stomach, and it didn't work anyway. I have had acupuncture but that didn't work. Along the way the doctors have given me a few Hydrocodone and Oxycodone prescriptions, and sometimes I get them when I go to the Emergency Room. They hardly make a dent in the pain, but they are better than the over-the-counter drugs I have been using.

That is where I was until about six months ago. My girlfriend, Joan, and I were out with friends, and I had one of my headaches. So there I was making a pretty unpleasant scene, banging my head against the wall with the right side of my face red and my eye congested like pinkeye. One of our friends was using Methadone for her back pain, and she suggested I try it. I couldn't believe what happened. It didn't take more than 20 minutes. My headache went away, and I had a sense of calmness that lasted the night and into the next day. Twenty-four hours without a headache for the first time in over a year! What's more, my bipolar disease was better. I didn't feel nearly as nervous and angry as I usually do.

My friend has been sharing her Methadone with me. I will get 20 or 30 pills a month and use about three a day, and I will have one good week a month. I will be very honest with you, Dr. Cochran. I do purchase the Methadone off the streets when it is available, and that is not much. I talked to my doctor about it, and I was totally honest with him, but that was probably the worst mistake I have ever made (and I have made lots of them). He told me I was drug-addicted, that I had analgesic rebound headaches, and it was illegal for him to prescribe Methadone. I had discovered your Web site by then, and I asked him to look at it. He refused. Instead he gave me the drug, Suboxone, which, I am sure you know, is supposed to prevent cravings for opiates. It is important for you to know this, Dr. Cochran. I wasn't craving the Methadone. I was only craving some relief, and Methadone gave that to me. But he wouldn't listen. I took the Suboxone for a few weeks, and it did nothing except label me in my community as an addicted drug seeker. I live in a pretty small town, and every doctor here knows about me and the emergency room also. They used to be pretty nice when I went in there for a headache. When I have to go now, they don't treat me with much respect, but they will give me some intravenous opiates until the headache gets better.

Now about my bipolar disease. My moods change depending on the circumstance. I have a tendency to become extremely angry and violent, sometimes hitting people. I was always fighting when I was growing up. I also feel very nervous and worrisome. I think sometimes I am a hypochondriac. I am depressed, and I have no interest in activities I used to love, martial arts, guitar, drums, singing, sports, or just spending time with Joan and her children. Mostly I am angry. People are scared of me. My mother has been telling me how she sees an empty, hateful, violent shell that once was John.

Here is a little bit of history. I was born in 1979 and grew up with a mother and stepdad who gave me no acknowledgement. I was in trouble in school and ended up having to be removed from one middle school and sent to another with a second chance program. This was because of my behavior, not my brains—I am extremely smart. After high school I got into trouble again and went to jail for three months. After that I met Joan and moved in with her and her daughters. Eventually after losing several jobs due to my bipolar disease and anger, I started my own painting and drywall company. I was near great success when the chronic cluster headaches hit. Ever since then I have been searching for a doctor that knew or would listen to the facts I had come to know. And now you, and that is where I am at. Your Web site has given Joan and me some hope. I believe your thinking is correct. There is no way that my recovery from the Methadone could be a placebo effect or some kind of product of my imagination. If you will accept me as a patient, I will come to Tennessee. I don't have any money, but my brother says he will help me get down there. I desperately need help, and I am sure that if it is not forthcoming, I will commit suicide. It is against my religion, and I certainly don't want to do it, but the pain is unbearable, and my life is empty. I am no good to anybody.

God bless you Dr. Cochran for reading this. I look forward to hearing from you.

John Reynolds

I saw him in the company of Joan. She was quite pretty and half a head taller than John, who was short of stature and wiry of frame. He had a narrow face with close-set eyes. His hair was cropped short, and he exuded animal energy.

"John, I have gone over your e-mail several times. Let me compliment you. It is very well written and very descriptive. You have given me a lot of very valuable information, and we need to discuss it."

"Sure, I'll tell you anything you want to know. You are my last hope."

"Tell me about your childhood. What was it like?"

"Not very good. I wasn't very happy as a child."

"Was there abuse?"

"Not really but, well, maybe some verbal abuse. My parents were always fighting, and for that matter, my whole family, uncles, aunts, and cousins were always angry and fighting with each other."

"And then problems in school—tell me about that."

"When I started middle school, I had lots of friends. I got along with everybody, and everybody liked me. But then I started getting in trouble.

Like I wrote you, it wasn't my brains that gave me trouble, it was my behavior. I was always angry and ready for a fight. That is why I got transferred to another school."

"Did you graduate from high school?"

"No, I left after the eleventh grade. I just couldn't seem to get along with anybody."

"And then you were in jail for a while—tell me about that."

"It was a burglary."

"Why?"

"I don't know. I sometimes do things that I know are wrong, but I just can't control it. Same way with my anger. That's part of my bipolar disorder, isn't it?"

"That is correct. Now, John, you were diagnosed with bipolar disease maybe twelve or thirteen years ago. I suppose you were being seen by a psychiatrist?"

"My doctor told me I was a manic-depressive. I went to a psychiatrist and was given lots of different medicines, but none of them worked. A lot of them made me feel worse."

"Do you remember the names of any of the drugs?"

"Yes, a few. I remember Lamictal and Depakote and Prozac. Prozac made me manic."

"What is mania like, John?"

"Anger mostly, but also when I am that way, I feel hot, sweaty, and nervous."

"How long does it last?"

"A few hours or maybe even a few days."

"Do you feel depressed?"

"Yes, a lot. I have trouble sleeping, and I don't have an appetite, and I am really sad most of the time."

"Do you still see your psychiatrist?"

"No, after two or three years I gave up on psychiatrists. None of them were helping me. The only person who has really helped me and stuck with me is my counselor. I see him whenever I can."

"Tell me about your counselor, John. Is he or she a psychologist?"

"No, he is a social worker."

"You say he has stuck with you. What is he trying to do with you?"

"He is trying to teach me to control my behavior. He is trying to teach me how to keep myself from getting angry."

"Have you told him about the Methadone?"

"Yes, I mentioned it to him, but he said that he couldn't talk about that. He seemed a little bit put off by the idea."

"Tell me about the Methadone again, John. You said that the pain went away and stayed away for nearly twenty-four hours. Is that correct?"

"Yes."

"And you wrote in your e-mail that you felt calm, that you weren't angry or nervous. Were you feeing euphoria? Or an unnatural happiness?"

"No, I was more surprised than happy. It is hard for me to put this in words. I just felt even. I remember thinking to myself, 'this is the way normal people feel.'"

"And you have told your doctors about the Methadone?"

"Yes, I have several times. I hear the same thing from every one of them—that Methadone is not approved for the treatment of cluster headaches or bipolar disease—and they all refuse to give it to me."

"John, you commented about suicide in your e-mail. Have you ever attempted suicide?"

"No, but several months ago I was awfully close to it. I have a handgun that I keep locked up, but I was thinking more and more about suicide, enough to take the gun and put it on my bedside table to have it ready when I needed it. Dr. Cochran, you have to understand—I don't want to commit suicide. Joan and her daughters mean the world to me. My life is a living hell, but I love them deeply, and I want to live for them. I want to be able to provide for them, but my urge to commit suicide was becoming almost overwhelming. Joan called the suicide prevention center, and I was admitted to a clinic for a couple of days. They gave me some pain medicine for my headache, and I settled down. They discharged me and told me to follow up with my counselor. That is when we found your Web site, Dr. Cochran. You talked about Methadone being good for bipolar disease and also good for migraine. Joan and I are very hopeful that you can help me."

"Well, maybe I can, John. Maybe I can."

I was very taken with John. He had a remarkable ability to compose his thoughts and his words. There was an air of eagerness, hopefulness, and even confidence in his bearing. This, I must remind the reader, is often the bipolar way. When they are *euthymic* (normal mood), they can be quick, bright, and even commanding. That same demon that drives their emotional swings, when at least partially assuaged, renders them creative and able, and many bipolars live lives of great achievement.

John's story is a testament to the relationship of pain to bipolarity and testament also the remarkable benefits that can occur with opiate therapy.

In this book I will return to several of the themes presented by John, so I want to review his history in some detail.

The predominant, and most destructive, of his bipolar symptoms was a penchant for anger. I will advise the reader that this is a common bipolar symptom and advise also that it is only a minority of bipolars who experience the classic mood swings between suicidal despair and grandiose euphoria and disinhibition. John's description is rather typical. With mania he felt angry and also "hot, sweaty, and nervous."

His disease first exhibited itself as juvenile misbehavior, and it took a few years before the underlying bipolarity was recognized and treated, albeit unsuccessfully. Interestingly, those drugs, the mood-stabilizing anticonvulsants, which are used for the treatment of bipolarity are also, as I have mentioned, useful for the prevention of migraine. In John's case, they helped neither disorder. I want to introduce an idea briefly mentioned in the introduction that I will return to frequently throughout this book. That is, migraine in the bipolar is a often a very severe disease, unresponsive to conventional therapy, but frequently responsive to opiate (or stimulant) therapy.

John ultimately gave up on his psychiatrists, and this, also, is the bipolar way. Frustrated by repeated failure of treatments, they abandon their physicians and struggle as best they can with their unstable moods. Some learn to overcome, by force of will, their mood shifts and impulse, and that is what his counselor was trying to help John do. It works some of the time. Even the bipolar demon is subject to control by the better angels of our nature. But the capacity to control does not come quickly. It usually comes after years of destructive behaviors and their consequences that the victim realizes that he must learn to control his feelings and impulses.

His headaches began when he was quite young, and it does happen. Childhood migraine is not uncommon at all. And then, at age twenty-six, some four years before he came to me, his migraine changed into an even more violent form of pain—that known as cluster headaches. It is considered by most to be a variant of migraine. The name cluster derives from the fact that the headaches cluster in time. They are of brief duration, an hour or so, but they are intense, and they reoccur through the day and particularly the night. They may persist for weeks or a month or so and then disappear for months or even years only to reappear as before. An unfortunate minority of men with cluster headache (it is a male-predominant, almost an exclusively male, disease) suffer them incessantly without respite. This condition is the awkwardly named chronic cluster headache. It is without question one of the most distressing painful disorders there is. It was in John. As he wrote me, his headaches were occurring eight times daily. And then relief, blessed, miraculous relief with the opiate, Methadone.

A slight digression here. We physicians admonish our patients to take our prescriptions as ordered and under no circumstances to share the medicine with others. Nor, they are admonished, are they to take medicines that are prescribed for others. The sharing of drugs is not only illegal, it is potentially dangerous. Nonetheless, we have to accept the fact that people do share pills with each other. Sometimes, I suppose, it is simple curiosity, but sometimes it is an act of desperation in the recipient and an act of compassion in the donor. I can't endorse the practice, but I accept that it happens a lot, and it can lead to important discoveries. It certainly did with John, and it has done so in others that I write about.

I must ask you what would you have done if you were in John's shoes? Depressed, mood-unstable, angry, bitterly painful, and then the discovery of a cure with borrowed Methadone. Let's give John credit. He was honest with his doctors. He told them that Methadone was the only drug that ever helped him, and he requested their assistance. His request was treated with the response that it would be illegal to treat cluster headaches or bipolar disease with Methadone.

It is really not illegal at all! Look at it this way; John's friend, the one who shared her Methadone with him, was given that drug legitimately and legally for her backache. Why could not John have been given Methadone for his headache?

The cluster headache is one of the most vivid syndromes in all of neurology. The painful eye is swollen, reddened, and tearful. A clear discharge drips from the nostril on the same side, and sometimes the eyelid is drooped and the pupil constricted. It is easy to diagnose if the right doctor sees it during an attack. And that doesn't happen very often. And this brings me to an important point about the cluster headache. I doubt that many neurologists would contest my statement that one of the defining features of the cluster headache is that it is almost always misdiagnosed at first. It was in John and with unfortunate consequence.

His headaches were first thought to be due to a sinus infection. This is understandable for the symptoms of cluster and sinusitis are similar and, curiously, cluster headaches often have a seasonal incidence—thus the suspicion that the headache is due to allergy and sinus trouble. He did not, however, respond to appropriate therapy. This spanned an interval of a couple of years during which time he had his molar teeth extracted and then was given of a dental guard. He also submitted to acupuncture. During this time, his request for painkilling drugs and his visits to the emergency room were becoming more and more frequent. Misdiagnosis continued. John was judged to have *analgesic rebound headache*. That is, he was having headaches because of the various pain medicines he was taking. He was told that his headaches would go away if he quit taking pain medicine! I have written extensively about the analgesic rebound headache. I abhor the term and the mindset that generates the idea that a person's pain will go away if he simply quits taking the pain medicine. It is an exercise in magical thinking that, in my experience, never works.

And then, some six months before coming to me, the providential discovery that Methadone would not only relieve the pain of his headache, it would, if taken regularly, prevent the headache from occurring. Moreover, it greatly relieved his anxiety and anger. John reported this unlikely scenario to his physician. He was judged to be drug-addicted. His doctor prescribed Suboxone to diminish his cravings. Unfortunately, the drug did nothing for John except label and stigmatize him as a hardcore drug addict.

I was accepting of John's history in its totality. There were absolutely no loose ends. Everything he told me fit with what I had learned of pain, bipolarity, and the opiate cure. I was willing to write a prescription for Methadone. Hopefully, I could, in correspondence, convince his physicians in New Hampshire that opiate therapy, however unconventional, was appropriate.

I gave John a prescription for Methadone, 10 mg three times daily, one month's supply. He was to call me in three weeks and report his progress, and if appropriate, I would mail him another prescription.

John thanked me, and as he was preparing to leave, told me that his trip to my city was the first time he had ever been on an airplane. His greatest fear, he said, was that he would have a headache on the airplane and make a scene. Fortunately that didn't happen and now, armed with Methadone, it would not happen on the flight home. I then dictated a letter to John's physicians outlining his history as given to me. I reported on my own experience with the use of opiates, particularly Methadone, in the treatment of the bipolar in pain and included a galley proof of the chapter entitled "The Opiate Cure" from my soon-to-be-published *Curing Chronic Pain*. I enclosed copies of reports in the medical literature on the mood-stabilizing and antidepressant effects of the opiates in persons with bipolar disorder. (Admittedly, there are not many, but there *are* some, and that is very important.) I requested their assistance in providing opiate therapy. If they were unable to do so, John would have to return to see me every three months or so.

My subsequent office notes:

5/14/08. Phone call. He is doing fabulously well. He is able to work pretty regularly. Mood is better. Still having anger problems and still having headaches, but they are diminished. He is excited about seeing his counselor soon. I told him that I would mail another prescription for Methadone, going up to 20 mg three times daily from his current 10 mg. Call again in about three weeks.

6/10/08. Phone call. He continues to do well. He says, "I am a normal man again." He has got a full-time job. He is enjoying Joan and the kids a whole lot more. He still can't find a physician to prescribe Methadone. I told him to keep trying, and that I would send him a prescription for another month of Methadone.

7/10/08. Phone call. He sounds great. Still hasn't connected with a doctor up there. I will send him another month of the Methadone. Then if he hasn't found a doctor, he will have to come down here again. He did tell me that he was working regularly for a painting contractor, and that he had to take a drug screen. It was positive for Methadone, and he was referred for a physician's evaluation. John was able to present his prescription bottle, thereby validating that his Methadone was legitimately prescribed. He was able to keep his job.

8/10/08. First visit back, and he is doing splendidly. His counselor has been extremely helpful to him, and he has an appointment to see a new physician, primary care, and also an appointment to see a new psychiatrist. He has had good control of his bipolar disorder and migraines. He does have a little headache on awakening in the morning, cluster-type, and also an occasional migraine, but he is vastly improved. He volunteers that he can certainly see himself in a much different light and a much better light than before, and he realizes he will have to make some personal adjustments to try to control his anger, which has been a huge issue for him. This man has made enormous strides. He is currently taking 20 mg of Methadone three times daily. I am giving him license to go up to 30. He will call in a month or so, and I will mail him another prescription. Maybe the increased dose will help control his anger, but I very much want him to start getting his Methadone from a physician in his community. It certainly has been a life-restoring drug for him.

John and I remained in contact by phone and e-mail for the next several months. He told me it was impossible to find a doctor who would prescribe the Methadone. Maybe so, or maybe he was just tired of trying. He told me he was willing to accept the expense of traveling to see me every three months. It would be easier now that he had a job.

I saw John, in the company of Joan, when we were nine months into treatment with Methadone. He was working regularly, and I was satisfied with his compliance in taking my medicines. He did tell me that on several occasions he had to take extra Methadone because of his headache. This would leave him short a day or two before he could get his next prescription filled. He chose on those days not to work—fearful that his rage and anger would surface. I increased his dose to 40 mg three times daily and told him about the remarkable coincidence that this visit was scheduled on the date of my first book signing for *Curing Chronic Pain*.

"I am coming, Dr. Cochran. No way I am not coming."

"Where are you staying, John?"

"Near the airport."

"John, I appreciate the thought, but the book signing tonight is on the other side of town. Unless you have a rental car, the expense of taking a taxi will really be quite high."

"No matter. I am coming."

My signing was at a suburban Barnes and Noble store. I was discussing my book and answering questions when John appeared, Joan at his side. They stood at the back of the room, and he was smiling broadly at me. The discussions and questions and answers continued, and I kept glancing at John. By hand signs, he indicated that he wanted to appear before the group. I invited him to come forward and introduced him as an example of the opiate cure. He spoke for about ten minutes. I marveled once again at the presence and sense of command possessed by my young patient from New Hampshire. His words were chosen and offered with care but without hesitation. He recounted his history of bipolar disease and cluster headaches and also his misdiagnoses and mistreatment, this without bitterness or rancor. Then through tears, he told of his recovery and of the doctor who was willing to believe him. When he finished, there was not a dry eye in the house—not one, and that includes me.

I surely didn't want to follow an act like John's, so I moved away from the lectern and began chatting with some of the attendees, in effect concluding the presentation. Still, I was pleased to see that the crowd just couldn't get enough of him. They had to talk with him and even touch him. He was the absolute center of attention, and he was handling himself with grace, dignity, and good humor. It is the bipolar way.

Dr. Cochran:

I found your blog while searching for information on depression and opiates. I am 22, and I have suffered from severe depression and anxiety for most of my life. I have been diagnosed as bipolar, and I am currently taking 100 mg of Lamictal daily along with 1 mg of Xanax twice a day. I have been on the Lamictal for a month, and I haven't seen much of an improvement. The depression is still there, and it just seems to be getting worse. I am getting to the point where I can't take it anymore. I am in extreme mental pain on an almost daily basis, and I can't continue to live like this. I don't know what to do anymore.

During the past seven years I have tried the following medications: Cymbalta, Effexor, Zyprexa, Prozac, Paxil, Wellbutrin, Celexa, Lexapro, Elavil, Trazodone, Seroquel, Adderall, Strattera, Dilantin, Provigil, Ativan, and Klonopin. I feel like a lab rat, and most of these meds just made me feel worse. A few of them made me suicidal, others made me manic, and some just had intolerable side effects. Elavil seemed to help more than anything else, but it makes me feel drugged even at a low dose, and it doesn't completely get rid of the depression. It just makes me not care as much about anything, I don't want to live like that either.

My doctors would say that I have a history of drug abuse, but I would say that I have self-medicated because their solutions haven't worked for me. I don't take drugs for recreational purposes, I take them only to feel better. I have found two different drugs that worked very well for my depression. Unfortunately for me and others like myself, one of those is marijuana and the other is a class of drugs known as opiate. As you are well aware, neither is currently accepted as a treatment for depression.

But the fact is they both work for me, and they work with no side effects. They are like a miracle cure. They take away all my sadness, my anger, and my anxiety. They make me feel normal, and I am able to function. The problem is I can't get my meds from my doctor. She knows that I smoke pot, but I haven't told her that opiates help me because after hearing my drug history, she told me specifically that if I had a migraine to take Tylenol for it. Now I am scared to talk to her about this as I think she will probably just attribute my depression to my "drug abuse." I considered that as well, so I quit smoking pot for several months, and I didn't notice any improvement in my depression, which leads me to believe that pot that is not the cause of it. Normally I don't take opiates on a regular basis, so I don't believe they cause it either. I am not using any other street drugs, and I don't even drink alcohol any more. My depression came before my drug use anyway. Even if my doctor believed me, I am not sure she would prescribe an opiate for depression.

Since I have no reliable source for my medication, I run out of it on a regular basis. This is when my depression is at its worse, and it is close to being unbearable. It is pure hell. I tell my doctor this, but all she can do is give me medication and tell me to hang in there for another month while we see if this one works. It never does, and it is the same thing with every doctor. I am tired of going through this, and I am tired of suffering when I know there are drugs out there that work for me and drastically improve my quality of life. It is very frustrating to know there is a cure for my illness, but I can't have it!

In the past I have taken several different kinds of opiates, and they all work perfectly as antidepressants. They work just as well as marijuana, only it is much easier to control my dose with opiates, and they are not completely illegal. When I take them I have no need for other antidepressants, and with the right dose I don't feel high or manic. I just feel normal, and I am able to enjoy my life and get things done. In your blog you wrote, "When the right drug kicks in, everything gets better." I can tell you from my own experience that opiates are my right drug. The only problem is finding a doctor who will prescribe them for me for depression and not write me off as a drug addict wanting to get high.

From reading your blog, I know that you understand, and that is why I am writing you. Is there anyway you can help me, Dr. Cochran? Would you be willing to treat me or refer me to someone who can? I live near Louisville, but I can drive to Nashville every week to see you if that is what it takes to help me get better. Or maybe you could talk to my current doctor about this. Maybe she would be open to treating me with an opiate if she knew it would work and that I am just not trying to get high. Please consider my request because I am running out of options.

Rebecca Porter

She was a tall, long-limbed young woman who presented a most unusual image. Her auburn hair, cut shoulder length, hung down from her scalp like a canopy. It covered all the features of her head and neck except her nose, which protruded through it. She kept her face lowered, and words came slowly to her. With her mother's help, however, I was able to gather a little more medical history.

Her depression and anxiety began at age fifteen. She was diagnosed with attention deficit disorder at age nineteen and bipolar disease at age twenty-one. For the attention deficiency, she had been treated with the stimulant, Adderall. She found that very effective in improving her mental focus and helping her depression, but the effect was short-lived, and when it wore off she would crash into a deep depression. I learned that she had been admitted to a psychiatric hospital on one occasion because of cutting herself. She told me that was a euphoric experience, a way to release the anger she so often felt. She ultimately gave up on cutting when it no longer helped to control her emotions. She found marijuana very effective in relieving her depression and anxiety, but after several months, the marijuana actually became depressant to her. She acknowledged that in the past she had briefly used cocaine and methamphetamine. Both made her depression worse. She had used several different opiates—some obtained legitimately for treatment of her low back pain and others off the street. I asked if she had ever taken Methadone, and she told me no.

"Well, Rebecca, you have given me a lot to work with. You do have a pain problem and have been prescribed opiates for this. This gives me the option of prescribing opiates for your pain, and hopefully they will control your bipolar disease. I do accept what you have told me. I have seen others whose bipolar disease can be controlled only with opiates. You must understand that I demand your absolute compliance. You must take these medicines exactly as I prescribe. Call if you have any questions, and come back to see me in three weeks."

I wrote a prescription for Methadone 10 mg three times daily. It was a low dose given to see if she could tolerate the drug. I believed then, and still do, that Methadone is probably the most effective opiate for the treatment of painful bipolarity, but there are times when it doesn't work and other opiates do.

I stood up and extended my hand to Rebecca. She accepted it limply without any words. Then her mother took my hand in both of hers and with tears in her eyes said to me, "Thank you so much. You have given us hope. It has been so difficult for me to hear her saying over and over, 'I want to die, I want to die, I want to die.'"

Once again I dictated a long letter, just as I had done with John but a few months before, outlining my thoughts to her doctor.

I thought a lot about Rebecca and her mother for the next several days. I thought about her strange appearance. I had spent some forty-five minutes with this young woman and not seen any of her facial features except her nose. I worried about her use of cocaine and methamphetamine, the recreational drugs that she had not told me about in her e-mail. She told me she had gotten opiates off the streets but acknowledged that her grandmother had given her some Codeine. I wondered about her parents' role in obtaining opiates for her. Who knows? I thought about her back pain, which it seems was of sufficient severity in the minds of doctors at walk-in clinics to prescribe opiates for her. She had, however, never addressed the issue of back pain with her primary care doctor or an orthopedist. In almost no circumstance would I prescribe opiates for a twenty-two-year-old woman for back pain that had never even been investigated with an X-ray. But back pain it was, and however peripheral an issue, it legitimized, at least temporarily, my opiate therapy. If what she told me was correct, and

I was sure most of it was, the prospect for control of her bipolar disorder was high indeed.

On her next visit, Rebecca's hair was brushed back a bit. I could see more of her facial features. She told me that she was feeling better emotionally, and that her back pain was much diminished, but she was having a problem with nausea and sedation on the Methadone. She could only take 10 mg twice a day, less than prescribed. I elected to rewrite the Methadone up to four times daily knowing that the common early problems with sedation, nausea, or itching with Methadone tend to abate as time goes by. I would let her find her own level somewhere between two and four pills a day. I was pleased to learn that Rebecca had seen her psychiatrist who, I was told, was very impressed with her improvement and quite taken with my letter and my ideas.

A few days later, I received a call from Rebecca's psychiatrist. We had a nice chat, and she told me that she was astonished at Rebecca's improvement and that she would be very supportive of my efforts with such highly unconventional therapy. I appreciated that because it doesn't happen very much. Most psychiatrists recoil at the notion that Methadone, a drug used to treat heroin addicts, could actually be beneficial for bipolar disorder.

Three weeks later, Rebecca returned. Her hair was brushed back even more, and she volunteered that she could now hold her head up and look people in the eye, something she had not been able to do for years. That positive sign aside, she was unable to increase her Methadone beyond 20 and occasionally 30 mg a day for she was having problems with sedation. Moreover, she was still having intervals of depression and pain, the Methadone notwithstanding. I elected to introduce a second opiate, Oxycodone, to be taken, 15 mg, four times a day.

Only twelve days later, I received a phone call from her mother saying that Rebecca was much improved on the Oxycodone. She was, however, taking it at twice the prescribed dose. I told her mother to have Rebecca continue that dosage but to come in and see me soon because her supply would soon be exhausted.

A strange clinical scenario was about to play out over the next eighteen months, so it is important that you know why I did what I did. To begin, we must accept the fact that Rebecca was better in many dimensions, first on Methadone and then with the addition of Oxycodone. A young woman who but three months before hid her face from the world with her hair had become able to look people in the eye and converse with them. Her pain was diminished, and her mood was stabilized. Nonetheless, the usage of my prescription was reckless and noncompliant. This was, in any sense, drug abuse, and I had grounds simply on the basis of her actions for discharging her from my care. Four or five years ago, I would have done that, but I am, hopefully, wiser and therefore more tolerant. I was quite prepared to increase the dose of her drug according to need and to go to high, even extreme, doses if necessary because I have learned that the dose of opiates necessary to control bipolar disease can be quite high indeed (although sometimes quite low). I have also learned that the bipolar in pain knows, far better than I, *the appropriate dose to control all their symptoms*. So I did not scold. I simply advised that she should continue the dose that seemed to be working well. After all, if she was truly abusing the drug, which should make her worse, why was she better?

On her next return, Rebecca, for the first time, was unaccompanied by her mother. She told me she felt well enough to drive the two hundred miles to see me. She was excited about her progress, and she looked it. She was smiling, animated, and like many bipolars who respond to opiates, she actually looked prettier. I wrote the Oxycodone in a very liberal quantity—telling her she could go up to twelve of the 15 mg pills a day. That was a total dose of 180 mg. I told her again that I expected her compliance.

She returned sooner than scheduled for she had again run out of medicine. She had been taking 300 mg daily, twenty pills rather than the prescribed twelve. Nonetheless, she looked ever better, and she told me, excitedly, that she was looking for her own apartment. Her recovery had been sufficient to allow her to move away from her parents' care. I told her I was happy with her progress, but I did scold. The escalation of the Oxycodone dose was much too rapid for my taste, and Rebecca was exhibiting some behaviors of concern to me. She was going to do it her way and not my way and that, I must report to you, is often the bipolar way.

I threatened to discharge her from my care if she continued to take these drugs in such a reckless manner. She promised to take the medicine as I prescribed and told me that her psychiatrist had prescribed the antidepressant, Wellbutrin, and she thought that was helping her. I encouraged her to continue it and return to see me in one month.

She had gone up to 360 mg of Oxycodone daily, twenty-four instead of the prescribed twenty pills. She told me she was the best ever. She was living in her own apartment and making plans to go back to school to learn ecommerce and Web site design. I scolded once again but not too hard and wrote her a prescription for 360 mg of Oxycodone a day.

On her next visit, Rebecca told me what I had hoped for and halfway expected. There had been no more escalation in drug dosage. She was quite happy on the Oxycodone 360 mg a day plus Wellbutrin and Xanax. She said that for the first time in seven years she felt "normal." I was thrilled with what had been achieved. The dosage was quite high, but my patient was doing well—extremely well—and that is always the final determinant.

Rebecca had, over the course of several months, increased, perhaps recklessly, her dosage of Oxycodone. Does that make her an addict? Probably not because almost by definition the addict is never satisfied. The addict always needs more. When Rebecca got to 360 mg of Oxycodone a day, she needed no more. She had reached the threshold that gave her control of her bipolarity.

It went nicely for several months, and then she surprised me again. She had decided that Oxycodone was no longer helping her, so she began taking leftover Methadone. She stopped the Oxycodone, cold turkey, without any adverse effects at all. Moreover, she was tolerating the Methadone in higher dosages without any sedation or nausea. I was not surprised that Methadone, a drug that had given her uncomfortable side effects but a few months before, was now taken without any problems at all. This can happen, and I believe it may be unique to Methadone, and I will return to the subject later. I was a bit surprised, however, that this young woman could suddenly stop 360 mg of Oxycodone a day without the least hint of withdrawal effects. Perhaps it was the Methadone, a drug that we know can prevent withdrawal from other opiates. I was taken with her report that the Oxycodone just seemed to quit working. I reminded myself that she was bipolar, and a curious feature of bipolar disorder is that drugs that relieve it for a while sometimes suddenly quit working. We generally think of this in terms of antidepressants or mood stabilizers, but why not opiates? Still, I was perplexed. I had never seen anything like this before.

She did well on Methadone for a matter of a few months and then came in to tell me that she had discarded it. She felt it was making her depressed, and she had resumed the Oxycodone, again with benefit. I wrote another prescription for Oxycodone at 360 mg a day. I was unhappy with the way things were evolving, but my patient continued to do well. I remained servant to that observation.

I saw her next, for the first time in a year, accompanied by her mother. Rebecca had really lost ground. She was tearful.

"I am so depressed! This Oxycodone is depressing me. The worst in a long time. I want to get off these medicines. I want to be like other people and not have to take pills. I don't want to take pills the rest of my life."

Mother said, "She tried to come off the Oxycodone, but I told her to take more of it. She has been taking an awful lot of it, and it is my fault. I encouraged her to do it."

"Are you still taking the Wellbutrin?"

"No, I stopped that a few weeks ago. I thought it was making me depressed."

"She wants to come off these medicines. Do you think she needs to be detoxed? Do you think the opiates are making her more depressed?"

"That's right, I want to be off the medicines, I don't want to take any medicine."

I told Rebecca and her mother that I didn't think that was the way to go—yet. I wrote another prescription for Oxycodone and also for Methadone, hopeful that the combination of the two would arrest her depression. They told me that she had an appointment to see her psychiatrist within a couple of days. I told them I would communicate with the psychiatrist.

I certainly didn't understand what was going on. Response to a drug and then, suddenly, no response to the same drug. It can happen, but I suspected there was more than that. I began to think that although I had largely controlled her mood shifts, anxiety, and pain, I had not controlled her bipolar-driven impulse, recklessness, and disinhibition. This is the capacity, common in the bipolar, to have an idea and act upon it without regard for the consequences. It is the bipolar way.

I called her psychiatrist a few days later to discuss recent events and was told that Rebecca had not shown up for her appointment. The psychiatrist was rather negative, telling me that Rebecca had always been a noncompliant patient—missing appointments and not taking medicines as prescribed. She had known all along that Rebecca was using marijuana and probably abusing the Oxycodone and Methadone. It was interesting to me that the psychiatrist who had been so supportive of my unconventional therapy had become so totally unsupportive.

At the time of this writing, I am not sure what will become of Rebecca. She has not returned for her appointment nor has she returned my phone calls. I believe that opiate therapy helped her enormously. I also believe that stopping her drugs was an act of self-destructive bipolar impulse. It is unfortunate, but it is inherent to the disease, and bipolars will, often repeatedly, discontinue the drugs that are helping them. It's the bipolar way.

CHAPTER 3

Cure and Denial

I will tell the stories of many people whose suffering has been relieved and whose lives have been restored because of my recognition of the bipolar spectrum and its enormous breadth and the opportunity that gives for successful treatment. Of particular interest to me, as I have been writing this book, is the review of the charts of people who came to me before I had any awareness of the bipolar spectrum and the opiate cure. It is frustrating to read of their struggles and my struggles as I attempted, often unsuccessfully, to control their pain. Finally, when I was able to give them relief, I realized that I was curing a disease state, that is, pain and the bipolar spectrum, that I didn't even know existed but a few years before.

Mary came to me on referral in 2003. She was forty years old and had suffered progressive back pain dating from an automobile accident seven years previously. She was taking Hydrocodone for pain and from her psychiatrist, Topamax, Geodon, Librium, Seroquel, and Lexapro for her bipolar disorder. She told me that with her current therapy, her moods were no longer shifting, but she remained sleepless and depressed. I learned that she had suffered a difficult childhood with parental neglect and a rape at age sixteen. In her twenties, she was a heavy user of marijuana and opiates obtained on the streets. She terminated that activity when she entered a very satisfying relationship. She had one child, a son with attention deficit disorder and, she suspected, bipolarity.

I found myself in a familiar stew, treating a bipolar with chronic pain. I did not want to intrude on the psychiatrist's care by introducing any more psychopharmaceuticals, for I knew that the possibility was great that in doing so I would make her worse rather than better. I elected to increase her opiate therapy by giving her an extended release preparation of Oxycodone. She did get a measure of pain relief. I didn't ask if she got any improvement in her mood on the drug, because at the time, I didn't know that was possible.

Over the next several years, I learned that hers was a seasonally cycling bipolarity. In the spring she would feel happier and have less pain. In the fall her depression and pain would worsen. A year and a half into her treatment, her pain became agonizingly severe, and I elected to add Methadone, 10 mg three times daily. Maybe a different opiate would help her pain.

She returned a week later. She was distraught. Her face and arms were bruised, and her left shoulder seatbelt abraded. She told me her car had turned over several times, that she had to be cut out of it, and that she was lucky to be alive. She spent several hours in the emergency room. Fortunately, X-rays were negative for fractures.

"Dr. Cochran, ever since that accident, I can't think, I can't remember. I have no mental focus at all. My pain is much worse. I am scared, really scared."

"Mary, you obviously struck your head and face with some force to have all those bruises. Did you lose consciousness?"

"I don't think so. Do you think I have some kind of brain injury?"

She was presenting me with a rather difficult clinical problem. Concussions, which are almost by definition associated with loss of consciousness, can certainly cause memory loss and lack of mental focus. Or was Mary perhaps experiencing some kind of emotional reaction to her injury? Or could she have acquired, suddenly, attention deficit disorder as a result of both emotional and physical trauma? (It could happen.) And then, an insight.

"Mary, did you take that Methadone like I told you?"

"Yes, exactly as you told me. I am still on it."

"Does the Methadone do anything for you for good or bad?"

"I don't think so."

"Did you feel any way impaired taking the drug?"

"I'm not sure. Like I told you, I am not remembering so well."

"Mary, you were on Methadone for a few days, and then you had an automobile accident, and now you can't think right and remember. We have to get you off the Methadone."

"Will that help my thinking?"

"I don't know, but it is something we absolutely have to do."

I performed a neurologic examination and found no evidence of serious brain injury. She was not complaining of a headache, which in this setting would have been a very ominous symptom. I concluded that watchful waiting was in order, and she would just have to put up with the pain as best she could until I saw her again. I had to satisfy myself that her faculties were going to return. Fortunately they did.

On a routine visit a few months later, I elected to obtain a urine drug screen to check on her compliance. It was appropriately positive for Oxycodone, negative for Hydrocodone, and positive for marijuana.

"Why no Hydrocodone, Mary?"

"Well I do take more of it than I should. I always run out of it a few days before I have an appointment to come in to see you, and that is why the test is negative."

"And the marijuana?"

"I am back on it. It helps my mood and my pain."

It so easy to be judgmental, particularly when one has the results of a urine drug screen in their hands. I elected not to go there. I have learned that much the most common explanation for a negative drug screen is not that the drug is being sold on the street or taken for some euphoric high. It is because those with pain often take more of the opiates than prescribed in order to relieve their pain. It is a very common behavior. And the marijuana? It can be pain-relieving, and this has been established beyond debate. Its prescription is legal in about one-fourth of the states, illegal in the others. Regardless, it is widely used by those who suffer.

I repeated the drug screen three months later. It was positive for Oxycodone, Hydrocodone, and marijuana.

Over the following months, Mary experienced an uneventful hysterectomy and the eventful birth of her first grandchild. She also experienced an episode of mania after she elected to discontinue her Geodon because of its expense. During her manic euphoria, she spent money that she didn't have, and even with resumption of the drug she was suffering mood swings, irritability, and increasing pain. I was far wiser now than I had been when I started taking care of Mary. I made inquiries that I would not have made before and asked if she suffered vivid dreams.

"Yes, they are very real to me, and I have a lot of them."

"Are you ever paralyzed or mute, unable to speak when you awaken from a dream?"

"Yes, that happens a lot."

"How is your memory, your mental focus? You remember after your automobile accident that you had a problem for a while with that."

"Oh, I can't concentrate at all. My memory is just terrible. Just like after the accident."

"How long has it been going on?"

"Ever since I was manic about a month ago."

"Mary, I am going to give you a new drug. It is a painkiller called Methadone. It can be very helpful for your condition. With luck it will help your pain and your mood swings and maybe also your memory. I am writing it for you one pill—that is, 10 mg—three times daily. I want to see you back in a month, and I want you to call me if there are any developments of concern to you."

Neither Mary nor I remembered that some two years before, she had briefly taken Methadone. It was three weeks, not four, when she returned, and she looked better than I had ever seen her. She was smiling, and she had quite a story to tell.

"Dr. Cochran, this is the best I have felt in twenty years. It is the Methadone. It is the best medicine I have ever taken."

"Well, Mary, it is obvious that you are better. You look ten years younger than the last time I saw you. Are you taking the Methadone as I prescribed?"

"Well, I started out taking one pill three times daily like you told me and nothing was happening, but at least I wasn't feeling any worse. So I decided, and I will ask you to forgive me for this, to go up to two pills three times daily, and I did feel a little bit better. Then one morning I took three pills at the same time, and within a few hours I could tell that something was coming over me. I felt happy. I felt focused. I had more energy. I actually was able to get out of bed and clean my house. I am sleeping better, and I am not having bad dreams. I am euphoric."

"That is wonderful Mary, but I have to ask you, are you manic?"

"No, this isn't mania. When I am manic I don't sleep. My sleep is wonderful now. What's more, I have reduced my Oxycodone dosage. I am having very little pain."

"Okay, Mary, I accept what you say. You have experienced the opiate cure. Methadone has relieved your bipolar disease and your pain. I think it will probably continue to do so, but we may have to make some adjustments in your dosages as time goes by. What dose are you taking now?"

"I am taking 30 mg twice daily, and I am out of it now since I am taking the bigger dosage. Will you write it for me?"

"Yes, I will."

"Thank you, thank you again. I never dreamed this would happen."

"Mary, I want to talk about something else. I understand that your psychiatrist is retiring. I am sorry because I have worked closely with him over the years. Let me ask you, has he seen you since you have been on the Methadone?"

"Yes, and he told me to keep taking it if it was working for my bipolar disease."

"Good for him. Do you have a new psychiatrist yet?"

"Not yet, but Dr. Goldberg gave me the names of a couple that I could go to. He told me they would be very good."

Mary has been on Methadone for nearly three years now, and she continues to praise it as the best drug she has ever taken for her bipolar mood swings. But, curiously, although Methadone has continued to control her mood shifts, it has become progressively ineffective for control of her pain, and I have had to increase the dose of Oxycodone. This can happen. I have patients who get mood stabilization with Methadone but not pain relief. In others, Methadone affords pain relief but no mood stabilization.

On a recent visit, Mary and I had extended conversation. We reviewed our time together and, the backsets notwithstanding, just how well she really was doing.

"Dr. Cochran, I think you will be interested in this. I have a sister who lives in Connecticut. She is bipolar, and she has had as much trouble as I have. Her psychiatrist recently started treating her with Methadone, and she is responding. Isn't that remarkable? Two sisters, both bipolar and both responding to Methadone."

"Yes, that is remarkable. Tell your sister that your doctor is proud of her doctor. I am glad he is willing to try unconventional therapy to help her."

"That leads me to a question, Dr. Cochran. You gave me Methadone for my pain and bipolar disorder. Dr. Goldberg told me to keep taking it if it was working. The doctor in Connecticut is using Methadone for my sister, and it is helping. But when I told my new psychiatrist that my bipolar disease had been cured by Methadone, he told me that was impossible. I didn't like him very much, so I changed and went to another psychiatrist. She told me that my recovery could not have been due to Methadone, and that I ought to get off of it because I was going to become an addict. What gives, Dr. Cochran? Some say it is good, and some say it is bad. What gives?"

Reader, it is now time to address an important issue relative to this book and my work. Although the appreciation of the bipolar spectrum as an entity is gaining purchase in the psychiatric community, the notion that its many expressions could actually be relieved by a drug like Methadone is unconventional to the point of heresy. It is a new idea, and new ideas sometimes suffer a long period of gestation. But the problem is not just that we are dealing with a new idea; it is that we are dealing with opiates, drugs that we have long believed have no purpose other than the relief of pain and, with that, the risk of addiction.

I was able to witness Mary's recovery and so was Dr. Goldberg. The two psychiatrists who followed did not actually witness it. They could only hear of it, first-person, from Mary. They chose not to believe. Their reaction, and I am trying to be even-handed about this, is an exercise in the psychological defense mechanism that we physicians so often find in our patients—denial.

We all employ it. It is the reaction of the man who experiences chest pain with exertion or the woman who finds a lump in her breast. The consequences of these observations are unconscionable. It shouldn't be. It can't be. It is not—denial. The same with the opiate cure. Its consequences, the liberal prescription of addictive opiates to the mentally ill, is unconscionable. It shouldn't be. It can't be. It is not—denial. Faced with an improbable miracle, we enter denial. It happens to the best of us, even psychiatrists.

Laurel was forty-three years old. Her back pain began some fourteen years before. No certain cause could be found, and she was treated with spinal injections and physical therapy. She was taking Hydrocodone in small dosage.

She began seeing a psychiatrist for anxiety and depression some eight years before. When he recognized her bipolarity a year or two into treatment, he started her on Trileptal, which, she told me, was helpful for stabilizing her mood. Nonetheless, she experienced two intervals of suicidal depression, one with an overdose of Imipramine requiring two days on a ventilator. She acknowledged sexual abuse from age six to nine at the hands of her half brother. She remained in counseling for that. She had taken many drugs, among them Prozac, on which she became quite paranoid. She continued to flash back to childhood experiences and was on Xanax for anxiety. She was also taking Effexor. I prescribed Methadone in the usual dosage, 10 mg three times daily, and made sure to copy my consultation note to her psychiatrist. I wanted him to know.

She returned at the appointed three weeks to tell me she had had remarkable improvement in pain and also a sense of what she called "euphoria." She felt less anxious, and she needed less Xanax. She reported that her mind was clearer, and that she could think better. Although energized, she was sleeping much better than she had before, a clear sign that she was not manic.

Over the course of several months, I increased her dose of Methadone, and she did indeed become a bit manic, talking loudly and rapidly and spending sleepless nights cleaning her house. I reduced the Methadone and remained in communication with the psychiatrist. He appropriately increased the dose of Trileptal. Laurel did well and for many months we had a high level of stability on Methadone, Xanax, Trileptal, and Effexor.

"Dr. Cochran, have you been telling Dr. Jenkins about the Methadone?"

"Yes, I've copied him all my notes."

"Well, I am not sure he has been reading them. I saw him recently and talked about the Methadone with him. I told him it was the best drug I had ever taken for my bipolar disorder. He seemed to get angry. He said he didn't want me taking Methadone for bipolar disorder. He said there was no place for it in the treatment of bipolarity, and that it was a dangerous drug, that it was addictive."

"Well, Laurel, I am a little bit surprised at that. He sure knows what I am doing and what I am thinking—at least he should know."

"Well, no matter, I talked my way out of it. I told him you were giving me the Methadone for pain and not for bipolar disorder. He seemed to settle down after that. He was less confrontational."

Laurel continued to remind me on every visit that the Methadone had changed her life. But then a problem. Her psychiatrist left practice, and she was forced to seek her care elsewhere. She found a community mental health clinic. They were, she told me, reluctant to treat her because she was on Methadone. She told them that it had been very helpful to her, but they were disbelieving. They did maintain her Trileptal but told her they would not give her Xanax because of a potential interaction with Methadone causing respiratory arrest and death.

Well, it can happen, but probably not much if the dosages are closely monitored. She had been on the combination for a couple of years with no problem. And her electrocardiogram, which can often predict problems with Methadone, was quite normal. I took over writing her prescriptions for Xanax.

On a recent visit I asked her about an issue that is becoming increasingly important to me. That is the relation of childhood abuse to chronic pain and bipolarity. She informed me that since the Methadone, her flashbacks had diminished greatly, and that she had found herself just not thinking about her childhood as much.

Reader, please savor this. Methadone had relieved her post-traumatic stress disorder and its disturbing flashbacks—something that Xanax, Effexor, and Trileptal had been quite unable to do.

Now back to her psychiatrists. Were they in denial? Even though she told them the Methadone had cured her, they chose to disbelieve, as if believing the patient is important.

Marissa was fifty, facially scarred from burns at her age eight. She grew up, she told me, in a loving, nurturing environment. She had accommodated to her disfigurement, married, and raised three children.

Painful facial burns at age eight. A long convalescence with skin grafting. Disfigurement. Does that count as childhood trauma? Does that account for the subsequent development of anxiety, chronic pain, and, ultimately, bipolar disorder? One wonders.

Her bipolarity erupted at her age forty when she required hospitalization after a suicide attempt. She was to remain for ten years under the care of a competent psychiatrist. Along the way she was given the mood-stabilizing anticonvulsant Lamictal, which produced a rash—a sometimes fearsome consequence of the drug. Later Lithium, which worked well for several years. Xanax, given for anxiety, induced mania (it can happen). It was replaced with Klonopin, which she found agreeable. When she came to me she was taking Cymbalta, Klonopin, and the sleeping aid, Ambien.

She described her manic episodes as "a whirlwind in my mind." She would become agitated, angry, sleepless, and unable to think or concentrate with these episodes typically lasting several days to a week. Depression remained her predominant symptom until several months before coming to me when she developed intense pain in her neck, arms, and hands. Ruptured discs were found in the neck. They were compressing the nerves of the upper extremities, and she underwent surgery to stabilize displaced vertebrae. Pain was diminished for a short while, and then it reappeared, prompting her referral to me.

Her new pain was confined to her hands, which were numb and burning. She was taking Hydrocodone in a low dosage, 5 mg twice daily, given by her neurosurgeon. Each pill gave her about two hours of relief. I elected to start with Methadone because, as I have certainly indicated, it can be uniquely beneficial for the bipolar in pain. I copied my consultation note to the neurosurgeon and to the psychiatrist who had cared for her so diligently and had even sent me a letter introducing her.

Her response was quite favorable. She told me that with Methadone she felt an emotional evenness that she had not known for a decade. Her pain, however, was in no way relieved.

Once again, Methadone controlled mood but not pain. This brings up an important issue. It is convenient to believe that those in pain suffer from depression *because* of the pain, and that relief of pain will obviously cure depression. It doesn't always work that way. I believe that we are depressed *as* we are in pain, not *because*. Pain and depression run on parallel but separate tracks, each subservient to brain mechanisms that are unique although often interdependent. I had controlled Marissa's mood but not her pain. The first order of business was to increase the dose of both Methadone and Hydrocodone.

Time went by and Marissa continued to extol the Methadone, but her hand pain was becoming ever more severe. Not unexpectedly, she began to question the use of Methadone. She had learned from friends, the Internet, and perhaps her psychiatrist that it was a dangerous drug and one capable of causing addiction. I tried to allay her fears by telling her that when a drug does what it is supposed to do, in her case relieving mood shifts and depression, that addiction was quite rare. And I meant it. I don't see addiction when the drug is working well. I see addiction when it is not working so well.

Marissa was found on *nerve conduction study*, the measure of the velocity at which nerve impulses travel, to have the *carpal tunnel syndrome* in both hands. She was scheduled for surgery to relieve pressure a nerve in her hands. I told her it was fine to pursue the operations, but I saw red flags waving. Think about it. She had hand pain as well as arm and shoulder pain from ruptured discs in the neck. Surgery had given her but a few months of respite, and then her pain recurred. Now she had a totally different disease—pressure on a nerve in the hands. She had not recovered from her neck operation. Would she recover from her hand operation? Moreover, why should she develop two unrelated disorders to explain the same symptoms? And why did they appear but a year apart from each other? How much of the hand pain was the residual of her nerve damage in the neck, and how much was due to nerve damage in the hand? How much of this was mere coincidence? How much was dictated by some higher force? And I am talking about her bipolar disorder.

The operations failed miserably. Her hand pain became worse. Even acts as simple as turning doorknobs was excruciatingly painful to her. She found that wearing heavy gloves was helpful to her. The need for heavy gloves notwithstanding, her mood remains stable. I added Oxycodone and made sure to copy my notes to her psychiatrist.

The Oxycodone worked rather well. It took a big dose, but Marissa was able to go without her gloves and open doors without difficulty. I was pleased with our progress. It had been obtained, however, at the price of aggressive opiate therapy in the form of Hydrocodone, Methadone, and Oxycodone. She remained, from her psychiatrist, on Cymbalta and Klonopin.

"Dr. Cochran, my psychiatrist thinks I am taking too much pain medicine. He says I am going to become an addict. He tells me he has drug called Sub-something, I can't remember exactly. He wants to use it on me."

"Suboxone?"

"Yes, that's it. Suboxone."

"So he wants you off the opiates?"

"That's right."

"Have you told him how much the drugs have helped you? Can he see that they have helped you?"

"I have told him over and over they have helped me. They have restored my life. I have my old Sissy back, and I want to keep her. It has been ten years, and I don't want to lose her."

"It is a free country, Marissa, you have the right to accept the form of therapy that you think works best."

Interesting to me that the psychiatrist who had witnessed a recovery from bipolar disease and pain with opiates had elected to terminate their usage. This was a treatment decision based, I suppose, on the potential harm from a drug against its proven benefit. Was the psychiatrist in some sort of denial?

Gladys Reasonover was twenty-eight when she came to me. Her back pain had begun at age eighteen and her anxiety and depression at age twenty-one. At age twenty-four her mood swings and attacks of rage were recognized as symptoms of her bipolar disorder, and her psychiatrist started her on Lamictal, Seroquel, and Klonopin.

A year before coming to me, Gladys was invited by family in Colorado to come for an extended stay. While there her back pain progressively worsened, and she sought the help of a physician. She was prescribed extended release Oxycodone and also marijuana, legal by prescription in the state of Colorado. She found the combination helpful. When she returned home, she went to a pain clinic where her Oxycodone was maintained, this for several weeks, until she was found on urine testing to have not only Oxycodone but also marijuana. She acknowledged its use to her doctors because, although illegal in my state, she was continuing to find it helpful.

From the pain doctor's office notes: "A urine drug screen was done, which revealed marijuana. I think Ms. Reasonover has a legitimate medical cause to have pain. However, I feel that she has high risk behavior and would be at high risk for narcotic therapy . . . . I did provide a Clonidine patch for withdrawal and told Ms. Reasonover how to taper off her medication. Again, I do not feel she is a good candidate for oral narcotic therapy. I do not feel that their benefit outweighs the risk."

Curious that doctors in two heartland states could see things so differently. One gave her Oxycodone and marijuana, and the other discontinued the Oxycodone because she was using marijuana.

During her weeks at the pain clinic, Gladys had also consulted a neurosurgeon. He found a ruptured disc on MRI testing and proposed surgery to her. Aware that she was receiving Oxycodone, he told her that he wanted her to discontinue that drug in favor of a less potent opiate, Hydrocodone. He wanted to see how much pain she was really having before he did an operation. Gladys told him about her discharge from the pain clinic, and he referred her to me.

"Gladys, I'm not sure exactly why your neurosurgeon wants me to prescribe Hydrocodone instead of Oxycodone, but I will comply with his request if that is what you want."

"It is very much what I want. I am excited about having an operation. I want to do it because I need it, and it is going to make me well. Can you prescribe Hydrocodone for me?"

"Yes. I am going to write it for you, 10 mg up to four times daily. I would like to see you back in two weeks."

When she returned, she told me that the Hydrocodone was helping her pain quite as well as the Oxycodone had done and that her mood was much better—that she wasn't snapping at people as she was wont to do. She told me she felt more "tolerant" and much less anxious.

"That's remarkable, Gladys. I can't say I expected that to happen, but I have seen this kind of outcome before. I am willing to increase the Hydrocodone if you think it would help you."

"Yes, let's go up on that. By the way, I am wondering if I want to go through with this operation. I am really not having much pain now, and my moods are better than they ever have been. My psychiatrist sees it. She is very pleased."

Gladys' recovery was an exercise in serendipity. I gave her Hydrocodone at her request and the request of her neurosurgeon. Left to my own devices, I would not have done so. If the Oxycodone was working, and it was in controlling her pain, there was no need to make a change. But in doing so, I had unwittingly controlled her bipolar disorder.

A short while later I received a fax from the psychiatrist.

> Dear Bob:
> I saw Gladys on November 2, and this is the best she has looked in a very long time. You have done a marvelous job with her on pain management.
>
> Lindsey Howell, MD

A very nice note and I appreciated it, but I wished the psychiatrist had been able to write, "You have done a marvelous job with her bipolar disorder." Maybe she was tempted but just couldn't do it. She witnessed the improvement, and to give her credit, she didn't enter denial. Unfortunately, however, she couldn't quite enter acceptance. Thus, the slightly disingenuous "You have done a marvelous job with her on pain management."

Jonah, age nineteen, experienced progressive low back pain. His orthopedist had performed the necessary obligations, which included physical therapy and spinal injections to relieve inflammation in the nerves leaving the spine. He did not countenance surgery in one so young and referred Jonah to me.

Bipolars live lives of great velocity. Jonah was certainly an example. He already had three children and had plans to get married soon. He worked on a loading dock but was on temporary disability because of his pain.

He was learning-impaired from early on, and a diagnosis of attention deficit disorder was made at his age eleven. He was given Ritalin but did not tolerate the drug. At his age thirteen, his grandfather died, and Jonah, grieving, attempted suicide. His bipolar disease was recognized, and he was started on therapy. As is often the case in the bipolar, several antidepressants made him more depressed, and a few made him manic. When he came to me he was on Xanax, Risperdal, Depakote, and Seroquel, and he told me his moods were in rather good shape on these drugs. He was taking Hydrocodone for pain, and he told me it was very helpful to him, that it energized him. He could do more when he was on the Hydrocodone.

The Hydrocodone-energizing effect is not uncommon. Indeed, many people have trouble sleeping when they are on the drug. Jonah was already on maximum dose, so I added Methadone, pleased that I had another opportunity to explore the effects of that drug in the bipolar in pain.

After only a couple of pills, he experienced nausea, dry mouth, sweatiness, and sedation. I tried Oxycodone, but that too was sedating. Next I tried Morphine. It was ineffective even in high dosage. Next was Meperidine, also ineffective. Jonah requested that we try the Oxycodone again. I did with the same results as before—sedation. Jonah more or less accepted his fate, that he was going to have back pain for the rest of his life.

I maintained Jonah on his Hydrocodone for several months and encouraged him to continue his psychiatric care. He did reasonably well for a while, and then, in an act of bipolar impulse, he decided that he didn't need his Seroquel, Risperdal, Xanax, and Depakote. He discarded them and in short order began to experience thoughts of suicide and also anger—this in spite of resuming his therapy. He consulted his psychiatrist and was advised to return to me to try the Methadone again.

"Dr. Robinson told me to come back to see if you would give me Methadone again. He said that sometimes people have trouble with Methadone at first and then get where they can take it. He told me it was a real good drug for bipolar disease, and he asked me to try it again. He wants you to prescribe it."

Remarkable! It was the first time a psychiatrist had ever referred a bipolar patient to me for treatment with Methadone. Remarkable also was his awareness that people who are intolerant of Methadone at first often respond quite well when it is reintroduced weeks or months later. It happens quite a lot (Rebecca in the previous chapter), and I have seen the effect with no other opiate. The psychiatrist knew at least as much as I did about bipolarity and the opiate cure, and probably more. I wrote a prescription for Methadone.

"It is the best drug I have ever had."

"Tell me about it."

"I am happier. I have more energy. My moods aren't swinging all over the place, and my pain is just about gone. I can put in a full day's work without hurting now. I can't believe how much better I feel."

"I'm happy for you, Jonah. Have you seen Dr. Robinson since you started the Methadone?"

"Yes, he is pleased."

"Anything else, Jonah?"

"Yes. I stopped the Risperdal and Depakote. I don't need them anymore, and I feel better off of them."

"Does your doctor know about that?"

"Yes, it is okay with him."

I don't know why it is, but things just seem to happen to bipolars. Jonah got married and the same day suddenly lost his other grandfather due to heart attack. Unsurprisingly, bipolarity erupted again with anger and mood shifts. His psychiatrist added Lamictal and requested that I increase the Methadone, which I did, and Jonah is stable once again.

I respect Dr. Robinson enormously. He has gone, it seems to me, where others have feared to tread. I find it interesting that the psychiatrists I have mentioned in this chapter, all of whom live and work within a few miles of each other, all of whom are on the staffs of the same hospitals, all of whom read the same medical journals, and all of whom, I suppose, communicate periodically with one another, have such divergent beliefs about the role of opiates in the treatment of bipolar disease. Hopefully, with time, we will all get on the same page.

I recently attended a national conference on pain management and had the opportunity to hear speakers discuss fibromyalgia. One of them, a rheumatologist, pointed out the frequency of bipolar disorder in those who have fibromyalgia. It was the first time I had ever heard any reference to bipolarity and pain in such a program. I was very taken by it, and at the end of the presentation I went forward to introduce myself to the speakers. I told the rheumatologist that my own experience was very much in line with the ideas that he was presenting. I also told him that I had many patients with pain and bipolar disease in whom both disorders responded to the administration of opiates, particularly Methadone. The rheumatologist's eyes got big, and the other speaker, a psychiatrist and pain management specialist, entered the conversation. "Yes, I have seen it myself."

My eyes got big.

"You have, you really have?"

"Yes. I don't know what it means, but I have seen it."

"Well I have seen it too, maybe dozens, if not a few hundred times."

"Have you really? Have you reported these?"

"No, but I have written a book about the subject, and I would like to send you a copy."

"Why, thank you. I look forward to reading it. We know so little about the effects of opiates on mental illness. I suspect there is something there that is very important."

"I agree."

The opiate cure is out there, and others are beginning to see it. Will it ever enter general usage? Will psychiatrists use drugs like Methadone for treatment of the bipolar? Probably so. It seems that is what the psychiatrist in Connecticut is doing for Marissa's sister and what Dr. Robinson wanted me to do for Jonah.

CHAPTER 4

Cure and Stigma

Harold was an interesting person. He was forty-two years old, tall, redheaded, and extravagantly tattooed. His face was spared of adornment, but no part of his extremities was unblessed. This was evident because he always wore shorts and sleeveless shirts, even in inclement weather. His voice was strangely nasal and high-pitched, and he had a peculiar behavior that I was to witness over the course of some ten years. During our visits, he would always position himself on the exam table, never in a chair, and would lie face up or curled into a fetal position. For many years I never had a meaningful conversation with him when both of us were upright. His speech and mannerisms notwithstanding, he possessed a certain charm, and he invariably flirted with my nurses, although never inappropriately so, and my staff and I came to enjoy his visits for he was certainly a break in the day.

He was married with children, and he worked as a meat cutter. Some two years before he injured his neck and required an operation. His neck and arm pain continued, however. He was given Hydrocodone and referred to me. He acknowledged sleeplessness and depression, and I prescribed for him my usual start-ups, Klonopin and Imipramine. Later, as I was preparing to dictate my consultation note, I reviewed the records of the referring doctor and saw that Harold had been abusing his drugs. I had not picked up on that but made a mental note to address the issue on his next visit.

He reported that he was feeling better. His pain had been at least partially relieved and his depression was also. However, I was to learn that was taking his Hydrocodone six times daily although I had written it for only four times. It appeared, indeed, that he was abusing the drug by taking it in quantities beyond what I had prescribed. This, I remind the reader, was over ten years ago at a time in my life when I was less than enthusiastic about opiate therapy. His overuse of the drug, the same behavior he had exhibited to the referring physician, was irresponsible and potentially a harbinger of addiction, and I told him so. Cautioning him against further abuses, I wrote another prescription for Hydrocodone, compromising with him and giving him five pills a day.

How foolish I was! Pain, as we all know, is a subjective experience, and there is only one person who knows how much pain he or she is suffering. The doctor really does not know and, therefore, must rely on the patient's report. So, the physician's dilemma—was my patient seeking something he didn't deserve, unnatural well being, or something he did deserve, relief of pain?

Harold got several months out of the Imipramine, Klonopin, and Hydrocodone, but then he relapsed. I liberalized his opiate therapy by adding Oxycodone, a stronger drug. Along the way I tried several other agents including anticonvulsants, always without benefit. Harold got by, but barely. I thought at the time that I had exhausted my resources, and there was no need for me to engage in exploring new options.

Some eight years into his treatment, he returned for a routine visit. I entered the examining room to find him supine, as always, but also bald. He initiated conversation.

"I've got cancer, Doc. I'm in chemotherapy," he said in his falsetto voice.

"Tell me about it, Harold."

"I had a lump come up in my neck. It turned out to be lymphoma. Here, look at my scar. I have just finished chemo. They tell me I am responding, but I don't feel very good. You can see how much weight I have lost."

"How are your spirits?"

"You guess. How would you feel?"

"I guess I would feel pretty discouraged."

"You've got it, Doc. I really am depressed."

"And the pain?"

"A lot worse."

I prescribed Zoloft and increased the dose of Oxycodone, believing at that time that I had nothing else to offer. Nonetheless, I scheduled a return in one month rather than the accustomed three.

He looked worse, not better. His tumor and his therapy had scarred his larynx, and his doctors had placed a tracheotomy tube into his neck so he could breathe better. He was unable to speak until he occluded, with his finger, the tracheotomy tube. Even then, his voice was only a high-pitched whisper.

With time, Harold stabilized. His tracheotomy was closed, and his larynx repaired to the extent that he could resume normal, if that is what you call it, speech. He continued, however, to exhibit sadness and hopelessness but all the while cracking little jokes and flirting with the nurses. On one occasion he told me that he had gone back to get his GED. He had never completed high school, never gone beyond the tenth grade. Seeking his degree was certainly a hopeful sign, and I encouraged him to pursue it. I told him I was very proud of his effort. I was to learn later that he just couldn't do it. He tried hard, he told me, but the academic work was just too much for him. What's more, his neck and arm pain had progressed to the rest of his body. It was, he told me, an all-over pain, a pain like no other.

"Harold, you have been taking Hydrocodone and Oxycodone for several years now. We do have more painkillers. Have you ever taken the drug, Methadone?"

"That is what they give heroin addicts, isn't it?"

"Yes, but it is a pretty good painkiller, and I am using it more and more. It just might help us."

"I am willing to try anything, Doc."

By this time in my care of Harold, I had witnessed the opiate cure several times, and I had learned that Methadone can sometimes be miraculously effective, especially in those who suffer from bipolar disease. I did not, however, put two and two together. I was simply trying another drug, hopeful that it might help my patient.

When Harold returned, I was shocked by what I saw. He was sitting upright in a chair and smiling. I took a chair facing him, realizing that for the first time he and I were not at right angles to each other. I knew something good was happening, and I couldn't wait to hear about it.

"How are you doing, Harold?"

"He threw his hands into the air and said, 'Thank you Jesus, thank you Jesus!'"

Pain is a subjective experience, and only the victim knows how much he is suffering. But not always. The physician may not know how much pain his patient has, but he often can tell when the pain is gone. Harold was a being I had not witnessed before. Even the pitch of his voice had fallen. I was elated.

"The pain, Harold, how is the pain?"

"Just about gone. I couldn't believe it."

"And your spirits?"

"Much better. I am hopeful now. Whoever invented that Methadone was a genius."

"How soon did you know the Methadone was working?"

"In a couple of days."

"Are you taking it like I told you to, a 10 mg pill three times daily?"

"No, Doc. I am only taking a pill and a half a day. It gives me a little nausea, but I am doing real good on what I am taking now."

Reader, let's reflect on this a bit. We know, don't we, that Harold was abusing his drugs at first. He was taking more than prescribed. Now he is taking less than prescribed. Is that also drug abuse? Let's give these people a break. They know what they need, and we should listen to them.

Then the inevitable question, because such a sudden and total recovery into wellness with Methadone occurs almost exclusively, in my experience, in the bipolar.

"Harold, we have never talked about this before, and we should have. It is my fault that we didn't, but has anyone ever suggested that you have bipolar disorder?"

He hesitated for quite a while and then said, "Well, yes, Doc. When they found my cancer, I was really stressed, and my moods were all over the place. Sometimes I would be agitated and really angry, and sometimes I would be crying I was so sad. The cancer doctor told me I had to see a psychiatrist before he started chemo. The psychiatrist said I had bipolar disease. She gave me some medicine to tame me. I guess that is the word, Doc, tame me, and I needed taming."

"Did the medicine help?"

"Yes, it did for a while. I don't think I could have gone through chemo without it. But after a while, it seemed to quit working, and I stopped it. I was still up and down until I got on the Methadone. That has been the best drug ever."

"I wish you had told me that before. It would have helped."

"Sorry, Doc, but I was ashamed of being bipolar. I didn't want you to know."

"Harold, have there been times in the past where your moods would swing, maybe times when you talked too much?"

"Yes, Doc, I have had it before. People would keep telling me to be quiet, but I guess I couldn't."

"Harold, you are bipolar, and that is probably why you have had so much pain for so many years. We have found a drug to help you, and it is helping you because you are bipolar. I am going to write you another prescription for it. I am writing six pills daily. I want you to listen to your body because it will, in time, know what the right dosage is. I am hopeful that the sense of nausea you have will go away. I think you will find that you will need more of the Methadone pills than you are taking now."

Harold is three years into his Methadone therapy now, currently taking 30 mg every eight hours, and I have been blessed to witness, with my own eyes, another resurrection of biblical proportions. Had I seen Harold three or four years ago rather than ten, my inquiries would have been directed toward the possibility of bipolar disease. I would have asked about mood shifts, agitation, anger, difficulty with attention and focus, and whether he suffered intrusive, unwanted thoughts. I also would have paid more attention to his tattoos. I do not offer a value judgment here, but I do think that extravagant tattoos can be a clue to bipolarity. Tattooing is a form of self-adornment, and that exercise, as in the wearing of brightly colored clothing and ostentatious jewelry, all the while exhibiting sadness, is a bipolar attribute. Also, Harold's capacity for simultaneous jocularity, flirtation, and sadness is, I believe, a bipolar attribute. The bipolar can be, and often is, both happy and sad at the same time.

Now I remind you again, did Harold have continued pain following a neck operation *because* he was bipolar? I suspect so. I believe Harold's chronic pain was an expression of his bipolar disorder—perhaps not the first expression, but the one that took him to a physician. Keep that in mind as you read the case studies that follow.

Jimmy came to me on referral from his neurosurgeon about ten years ago, just about the same time I saw Harold. He had been rear-ended in an automobile accident and suffered a whiplash injury with pain in the neck that persisted. The neurosurgeon could find little, certainly nothing to require an operation. He prescribed Hydrocodone and the muscle relaxant, Soma, and referred Jimmy to me.

I saw him in the company of his wife, both rather young people but clearly beaten down prematurely by circumstance. They were infected with human immunodeficiency virus (HIV) and were on treatment with monthly visits to an AIDS clinic for prescriptions and blood tests. Their disease had been acquired by intravenous drug use when they were teenagers, and they also carried the hepatitis C virus, similarly contracted. They were poorly groomed and somewhat unclean, but there was something about Jimmy that I liked. There was a straightforward earnestness about him, as if he was telling me that I was his last hope, and he would do anything I asked him to do.

He was depressed and sleepless, as they all are, and he told me that since his pain he had become moody and very irritable. In my ignorance at that time, I paid that no particular attention to that complaint. Just another victim of chronic pain, I thought. I maintained the Hydrocodone and also the Valium he had been on for several years. I added Klonopin and Nortriptyline. He did rather well. His pain was diminished to become at least tolerable. His sleep was much improved and his depression somewhat. Satisfied with what I had achieved, I elected to stay the course and arrange for him to return only every six months. It went well for a couple of years. He even became the singing director at his church, and he was quite proud of that.

Benefit was not sustained, however, and he required more and more drugs. I added Neurontin and then extended release Oxycodone, and with them, his pain lessened. His HIV infection remained in control although he did have several bouts of pneumonia. Over the years his opiate need escalated, and I added Morphine to his Oxycodone and Hydrocodone. I was more or less satisfied. He was by no means well, but at the time I felt it was the best I could do. Then a contretemps. His pharmacist called to tell me that he was receiving opiates from physicians other than me. His primary care doctor was prescribing a combination of Tylenol and Codeine, and it appeared Jimmy was taking on a regular basis.

On his next visit, I confronted him with my discovery. He hemmed and hawed as he searched for an answer. He told me that occasionally he has a fever and needs the medicine for that. Also, he said, his wife gets allergy shots, and they are painful, and she has to take one of his pills. Then he told me that he really didn't use the medicine very much, that he had lots of bottles of unused pills around the house. That struck me as absurd, and I was sure Jimmy was lying to me. Things were not going well for Jimmy because he also had to tell me that his last prescription for Morphine was left in his trousers when they were washed, and he needed a replacement.

I was being tested in a big way. His use of Codeine was in clear violation of his *drug contract* in which he pledged to receive opiates only from me. The lost-in-the-washing-machine story was one I have heard many times before. I accept it the first time, never the second, but the surreptitious use of Codeine was disturbing to me. It was a willful and deceitful act, and according to the terms of the drug contract, it was within my rights to discharge him from my care.

Reader, let's assume you are a physician. What would you have done? Remember, this man was an acknowledged drug abuser in his youth, and he was currently abusing drugs again. Would you have fired him? In quite ethically doing so, you could have solved your problem. How about his?

I don't know what it was that kept me from discharging him. Part of it was that I liked him a lot. I like his job as singing director at his church, his deceit notwithstanding, I liked his earnestness and his appreciation for my efforts. Perhaps more important, however, was his only modest use of Codeine. Two pills a day at most, and in relation to his other drugs, it represented a miniscule increase in his opiate therapy. I had become wise enough to realize that in the treatment of those in pain, justice must be tempered with mercy. I gave Jimmy and his wife a good scolding. I told them I wanted this to never happen again, and with that provision, I would continue their care.

On a routine visit a couple of years later, Jimmy had to tell me that he had run out of Oxycodone and Morphine before his next prescription was due. His pain had become intense and the opiates less effective in controlling it. He was taking them at twice the prescribed dosage.

"Jimmy, this is disturbing to me. I don't know why you should suddenly, after years on these drugs, be needing so much more to relieve your pain. Let me ask you, are you craving the Oxycodone and the Morphine?"

"No, Doc, I don't think so. Maybe I am craving them. I know I am craving pain relief. That is all it is, Doc. I just need pain relief."

"Jimmy, have you ever heard of Methadone?"

"Yes, of course. Everybody knows what that is used for. That is for addicts."

"You were an addict. Did you ever take Methadone?"

"No, I have never taken it."

"Well, Jimmy, Methadone can relieve the pain, and it is a drug I want to try on you. I am going to write you a prescription for it. It may agree or disagree, but I don't want any freelancing. If you have problems with it, call me, but under no circumstances do I want you to take more than I prescribe."

Methadone has the unique ability (along with Suboxone) to inhibit cravings for other opiates. Thus both can be used in the treatment of opiate addiction. We replace the drug that causes cravings with one that doesn't. In essence we replace a bad drug with a good drug. Another use for Methadone, which I employ not infrequently, is its administration simultaneously with the drug being craved. This usually inhibits cravings and in most cases provides additional pain relief. On top of that, if the user is also bipolar, that disorder can be very well controlled. It was to be in Jimmy. I wrote a prescription and handed it to him. Then almost as an afterthought, I asked, "Jimmy, has the diagnosis of bipolar disease ever come up with you?"

He paused for a long while and then said, "Yes, I was diagnosed as a manic-depressive when I was a teenager."

"Why in the name of God did you not tell me that before?"

"I'm sorry, Doc. I am ashamed of it, and I have always been. I just don't want to talk about it."

"Well, Jimmy, you are going to start talking about it now because it is very important. Tell me what happened to you."

"It was back when I was using drugs. I was depressed and sometimes I was manic. They put me in a hospital for several weeks. They gave me Lithium, and there were others."

"What others?"

"Well, I remember Haldol and Prolixin. I am sure there were some more. I was pretty sick for a while."

"Did you remain under psychiatric care?"

"Yes for a couple of years. I got off the street drugs, and then the Lithium and the others just quit working. I have lived with manic-depressive illness now for nearly twenty years, and I get by. My moods go up and down, but I don't think of suicide."

"Do you have any mania now?"

"Not really, mostly depression, but I did get manic on that Nortriptyline you gave me. I stopped taking it."

"Jimmy, that was several years ago! Why didn't you tell me?"

"I was afraid you would be mad at me. I was afraid you would fire me. I thought that if you knew I was bipolar that you would refuse to see me. Dr. Cochran, I've had doctors tell me they wouldn't treat me when they found out I was bipolar."

He was crying now.

"Jimmy, do you have dreams that frighten you?"

"Yes, I have had those all my life."

"Do they seem real to you?"

"Yes, very real. I wake up scared."

"Do you suffer from mind racing? Is your mind too busy? Do you have trouble turning it off?"

"Yes. I have studied about this a lot, and I wonder if I have ADD or something like that. I have always thought that Ritalin might help me."

"Well, it might, but we are going to try Methadone first."

"Thank you doctor. I will take it like you tell me. I think sooner or later you are going to get me well."

It was to be another resurrection. Jimmy told me that he felt better within a day or two. He was not, he said, as "foggy-minded" during the day. His mood shifts had lessened, and the Morphine and others seemed to work better in the presence of Methadone. His dreams were much diminished, and often their content was more pleasant. Even his opiate-induced constipation, a common problem, was reduced with the Methadone. As I have written so often before, when the right drug kicks in, everything gets better.

Jimmy has been on Methadone now for three years, and he, I think, enjoys the emotional catharsis of finally reconciling himself to his illness. He tells me, "I would never have asked for help for my bipolar disease. I was ashamed of it, and I think that depressed me as much as anything, even more than my HIV and hepatitis infections and my pain."

"I am happy for you Jimmy, really happy."

"Thank you, Doc, thanks for all."

What if I had fired Jimmy? Would he have ever found relief from his pain and his bipolarity? I doubt it. Treatment-resistant depression and treatment-resistant pain are strong indicators of bipolar disease, although I certainly did not know that when I first started seeing him. The administration of Methadone was an exercise in desperation—my willingness to try almost anything that might work. The dividends were huge, and I am grateful that I have had the opportunity to treat Jimmy and grateful also that I was able to cure, as with Harold, a disease that I did not know existed when they first came under my care.

Bipolar disorder is, in the minds of many, a shameful illness. It carries great stigma. Bad enough, but with the employ of opiates, particularly Methadone, a drug used to treat heroin addicts, the stigma is compounded.

Janet was a young musician with migraine. It had begun four years before with frequent headaches beginning in the back of the head and becoming generalized, although sometimes right-side-predominant. It was associated with painful sensitivity to light and sound, and she estimated she had a severe headache one day out of three. She also suffered pain in the neck and upper back due to fibromyalgia. As she became painful, she developed insomnia, depression, and anxiety. In desperation, she experimented with drugs including alcohol, cocaine, and marijuana, and found that these did relieve her anxiety and depression—at least for a while. Ultimately, within a matter of a few months, she realized they were making her depression worse, and she discontinued their use. She began to practice self-mutilation, cutting herself, an act that she said made her feel better, relieving at least for a short while her anxiety. Some two years before coming to me, she attempted suicide. She was admitted to a psychiatric hospital and the diagnosis of bipolar disorder was made. She began treatment with a variety of drugs including Lexapro, Seroquel, Lamictal, Ativan, and Klonopin. None were very effective, and as is so often the case, she abandoned psychiatric care. She sought pain relief here and there from physicians, walk-in clinics, and emergency rooms, and was occasionally given Hydrocodone and Oxycodone, which she said "made me feel normal."

"Janet, how are your moods doing now?"

"Not very good. I am up and down, and I hurt badly in my head and my back."

"What are you taking for pain now?"

"Nothing. I can't find a doctor who will give me pain medicine."

"You have a history of bipolar disorder. Do you get manic?"

"Yes, I guess so. I will have spells where I get very irritable and angry and, this is strange, if I go without sleep for a couple of nights, I become speeded up and agitated."

"What was your childhood like?"

"Well I thought it was pretty good although I remember I had night terrors, and I was also a very sensitive child. I have seen a psychologist recently, and she suggested that I might have been sexually abused. I have no memory of that, but sometimes I do wonder."

"When you take Hydrocodone or Oxycodone, it seems to help your mood?"

"Yes, quite a lot. I have wondered what that means."

"How are your memory and your mental focus?"

"Not good. I can't seem to keep my mind on any subject for any time. Sometimes when I am reading a book, I will come across a word, and it just doesn't register. I don't know what that means."

Janet suffered migraine and fibromyalgia. She was bipolar but unresponsive to treatment as so many of them are. Moreover, she was progressively inattentive and was having trouble with word recognition, which is suggestive of attention deficit disorder. I was taken with the fact that opiate therapy made her "feel normal." Interesting also was the psychologist's suggestion that there had been issues of sexual abuse.

"Janet, I am writing a prescription for Ritalin. As you may know, it is a stimulant, and I want you to be vigilant to the fact that it may make you worse. It may increase your nervousness, it may impair even further your sleep, and it may even make your manic. But there is an equal possibility, maybe even a greater possibility, that it will diminish all those bad things. I want you to be in close touch with me, and I will have you return soon for a follow-up."

Janet came back a week later with interesting information. She had taken the Ritalin and within an hour had an intense headache that pulsated and appeared in waves lasting a few minutes and then abating briefly but recurring. She had never experienced anything like that before. She did tell me that she slept very well that night, an experience she had not known for many years. That was certainly an encouraging report. I elected to discontinue the Ritalin and start a similar drug, Adderall, in very low dosage. I also gave her some Hydrocodone hoping that it would help her feel normal. She tolerated the Adderall and Hydrocodone quite well and had immediate relief of headache and for a while her back pain. Shortly, however, in a phrase she was to use frequently, she told me that she was "burning through" the Hydrocodone, and after two or three hours of comfort, she would get a headache and with it feel very angry. I increased both the Adderall and Hydrocodone. It didn't work. She kept burning through the Hydrocodone and perhaps, she told me, even craving it in an effort to get some relief. I told her to continue the Adderall and the Hydrocodone as before, and I gave her Methadone. Once again I was attempting to control both the pain and cravings with that drug.

On her return, she reported that she was much better. Her neck and shoulder pain was much diminished, and she was no longer burning through the Hydrocodone. She told me, with remarkable insight, that she was no longer obsessing about her pain, and that her mood was stable. Then but two weeks later, my nurse took a phone call. Janet had dropped all of her medicines down the toilet. I told my nurse to have her come in right away.

I was surprised at the story I heard. She recounted that with the Adderall, Hydrocodone, and Methadone, her migraines and fibromyalgia pain had disappeared, and that her mood was quite stable. In this state of wellness she was attending her sister who was giving birth for the first time. Janet went a couple of nights with limited sleep and then developed what was almost certainly an episode of mania. She became agitated and experienced thought racing during which time she decided that her medicines were making her worse, so she flushed them down the toilet. It was after a few days of opiate withdrawal that she decided to call me.

She and I had a long talk, and she told me that she wanted off the medicines. Also, for the first time, she informed me that she grew up in Minnesota near a methadone clinic. She saw a lot of unpleasant looking people there, and although the Methadone had been helpful to her, she was quite sure she did not want to take it anymore. I spent a long time telling her that she did not need to be off the opiates, that she needed to be on them, and that they had been curative for her. I told her that I understood her sense of fear, and that I understood the stigma that goes with taking Methadone. I told her also that she was not aligning herself with those who attend methadone maintenance clinics (not that there is anything at all wrong with that—they are only treating their illness), but I knew the stigma of taking Methadone was very real, and it was often a barrier to the successful administration of the drug. I wrote her prescriptions and urged her to resume her therapy. She told me she would.

We are now, at the time of this writing, over a year into Janet's therapy. She tells me she is happy, productive, and organized, and that she had her first date in eighteen months. She was also helping her sister through a divorce, an enterprise that would have been beyond her emotional resources but a year before. Still, she tells me, her recovery notwithstanding, she feels ashamed of taking the Methadone and has told no one but her father about it.

Patsy was only thirty-two years old but in pain for eight years. She suffered an industrial accident with injury to both shoulders that required surgery. She was left with chronic pain and an inability to raise either of her arms above shoulder level. She was ultimately released by her orthopedist to return to work but with restrictions including no overhead work and no lifting over fifteen pounds. Her employer told her that she could no longer work at his plant with those restrictions. She was fired. So, over the course of about eighteen months, she took a quadruple hit—injury, surgery, chronic pain, and loss of her job. Unsurprisingly, she became depressed and entered psychiatric care. Along the way she was given the antidepressant, Wellbutrin, which caused her to have a seizure and Prozac, which made her "absolutely crazy and headachy." Seroquel, the mood stabilizer, had done nothing nor had Adderall, which she said gave her headaches. When she came to me she was taking Zoloft, Xanax, and the sleep aid Rozerem from her psychiatrist and the muscle relaxant, Skelaxin, and Hydrocodone from her pain doctor.

Her psychiatrist was certainly being aggressive, and I respected that very much. She told me her depression was in fair shape, but her pain, the Hydrocodone notwithstanding, was really a bother. That was why the psychiatrist referred her to me for a second opinion.

"Did the psychiatrist tell you why he was giving you the Adderall, Patsy?"

"I think it was because of the depression. He says sometimes Adderall is a good antidepressant."

"Well, it can be. I'm sorry it didn't work, but let me tell you I applaud the psychiatrist for trying."

"Can you help me with this pain, Dr. Cochran?"

"Probably, Patsy, but a few more questions. How are you sleeping?"

"Poorly, I can't get comfortable at night because of my shoulder pain."

"Do you dream?"

"Yes, I have dreams, bad dreams—usually of somebody dying."

"Frightful?"

"Yes, quite."

"Do you ever awaken from a dream with a sense that you are paralyzed, that you can't move or speak?"

"No, I have never had anything like that."

"How is the depression?"

"It is not too bad. I don't think I am as much depressed as I am angry and irritable."

"Who are you angry at?"

She smiled and said, "Usually at whoever is around. I find myself snapping at my family and friends a lot."

"Do your moods shift? Are you up and down?"

"Yes, I am."

"What's up and what is down?"

"When I am up, I want to do things, I want to be with people. When I am down, I don't want people around me. I want to be by myself."

"What happens to the pain when you are down?"

"It gets worse."

"Patsy, has your psychiatrist suggested to you that you might have bipolar disorder?"

"No, but I think he wonders, and I wonder too."

"One last question. Does anyone in your immediate family have bipolar disorder or attention deficit disorder?"

"No bipolar, but my son has attention deficit hyperactivity disorder."

I was sure my patient was a "soft" bipolar, about which more shortly. I prescribed Methadone in the usual manner, 10 mg three times daily.

I enjoy my new patient consultations. I delight in the challenge and the opportunity that comes with new problems. Perhaps selfishly, I enjoy seeing people that other doctors have been unable to help, and that constitutes just about everybody in my practice. The visit that I anticipate the most, however, is the first return when I can see, usually when I enter the room, whether my medications are working. Since my discovery of the opiate cure, I often don't need to ask if they are better. I can see it in their eyes and in their expressions. Patsy was smiling at me when I entered the room, and I knew right away I had struck gold.

"Well, Patsy, how are we doing?"

"I can't believe it."

"How so?"

"The pain is gone! It is just about completely gone."

"I am happy for that, but I am interested in some other things also. Has anything else changed?"

"Everything has changed!"

"Tell me about it."

"I sleep through the night now, I haven't had a bad dream in the past three weeks, and I am calm for the first time in years. I don't feel irritable, and I don't feel angry. My family sees it. They are thrilled at what has happened."

"Have you seen your psychiatrist?"

"Not yet, but I am looking forward to telling him about it. Maybe I can come off some of this other medicine I am taking."

"Don't be too hasty on that. If you are doing this well, I suggest we not make any adjustments. By the way, how much Methadone are you taking?"

"I did just what you told me. I am taking three pills a day."

"Is that going to be enough?"

"I think so. I do have some questions for you, though. Will this last? Will I have to keep taking this medicine the rest of my life?"

"I don't know for sure, but the answer to both is probably yes, and I wouldn't be surprised if we didn't have to alter the dosage along the way. But in my experience, this kind of response is usually sustained. I am very hopeful for you."

"I am grateful to you, Dr. Cochran."

"I am grateful to you, Patsy, for the opportunity you have given me."

And I meant it. The joy, that dopamine moment of reward and gratification that comes with entering a person's life and relieving their suffering, both in their mind and in their body, is just about the most satisfying experience I have ever known.

Patsy's pain and depression have remained in control for several years now but, on a recent visit, "Dr. Cochran, I need a favor."

"Sure."

"My husband has filed for divorce, and I need a letter from you stating that I am taking Methadone for the relief of pain and not for treatment of addiction. There will be a custody battle coming up, and my lawyer tells me it is mandatory that I have a letter from you. If not, I will lose custody of my two children."

"I will write the letter for you, Patsy."

Jeremy was thirty-two years old. He was short, stocky, and stubble-bearded. His problems had begun some two years before when he had a sudden attack of numbness in his scalp and face and then high anxiety. He went to the emergency room, and a diagnosis of panic disorder was made. He was treated, I believe appropriately, with Xanax and Paxil. His panic attacks terminated, but he developed pain migrating from his head and neck into his chest and torso and then throughout his body. He became fatigued, and at the end of the workweek he would spend an entire weekend in bed to recover. He was found to have a ruptured disc in his neck, and he underwent, at age thirty, an operation. He told me that his pain and his headaches had diminished by some 50 percent with this. His improvement notwithstanding, he was unable to go back to work at the body repair shop. I was not at that time yet aware of the bipolar spectrum, and thus my inquiries were not as detailed as they have come to be. I surmised that his core disease was depression, the almost inevitable companion of chronic pain, and I prescribed Nortriptyline and Klonopin and maintained therapy with Oxycodone, Xanax, and Paxil given by his primary care physician.

A word now about *polypharmacy*, the simultaneous prescription of multiple drugs for the treatment of illness. It is a practice that is disparaged by some as excessive, and I will admit it does seem a bit untidy. Nonetheless, it is often necessary, just as it is in the treatment of diseases like hypertension and diabetes, and the bipolar spectrum with its attendant pain is vastly more complex than either of those.

Jeremy responded nicely. His pain was diminished and his sleep restored. Within but a few weeks he was back at work. After a couple of years, however, he began experiencing more neck pain and feeling more nervous. I observed that he was talking very rapidly and with a great deal of thought scatter. I made a few more inquiries. I learned for the first time that his mother suffered bipolar disorder. He also acknowledged he had been subject for a long time to intervals of depression. I increased his dose of Oxycodone, but it didn't go very well. On his next visit, Jeremy told me his wife wanted a divorce. I again observed his restless hyperactivity and very rapid speech. I prescribed Methadone.

It is interesting that Jeremy's illness had remained in control for a couple years on rather aggressive polypharmacy. And then, for reasons uncertain, it broke through and reappeared. This happens not infrequently, and the introduction of yet another drug or drugs is necessary. It's the bipolar way.

Jeremy loved the Methadone. He said he was relaxed with the drug, and that he felt calm and "even." A remarkable, almost universal statement of the bipolar when their disease is controlled is the use of descriptors like "balanced," "even," and "level."

Jeremy did nicely for several months, and then he reappeared before his next scheduled appointment. In those in pain, this early return usually indicates some problem with access to their drugs. It often is the result of overuse but equally often loss or theft of the drugs. The explanations I am offered are infinite in variety. In the main, I accept what my patients tell me. The worst part of the exercise, however, is having to listen to them explain in tedious detail the circumstances that led to the loss. Jeremy began by showing me a bottle full of several different kinds of pills. There was no prescription label on it.

"Dr. Cochran, you give me prescriptions for my medicines, I get them all filled, and then I arrange them in ten-day supplies. So each month I divide my medicines into three bottles just like this one."

"And?"

"I keep them at the very top of the medicine cabinet hidden in the back behind other bottles. I don't want anybody to know I have that kind of medicine in my house. I have to stand on my tiptoes to reach the bottles. I slipped, and one of them fell down. It hit the countertop, the cap came off, and all the pills rolled onto the floor. That's why I need more."

"Jeremy, I am accepting of what you tell me, but is there any reason you couldn't have picked the pills up off of the floor and put them back in the bottle?"

"No, Doc. No way. I will never put anything in my mouth that has been on the floor."

"Even for a few seconds? You could have picked up the pills in that length of time."

"No, I just couldn't do it, Doc. We have never talked about this, but I am a germophobic and a handwasher. I am sure I have obsessive-compulsive disorder."

It took me a little while to organize my thoughts, and then I asked him, "Jeremy, is that why you allot your pills in increments of ten days? Could you do it in increments of fifteen days or even one week?"

"No, that won't do. It has to be ten. Ten is perfect. The other numbers aren't. You see, I am a counter. I have to count out the pills exactly and place them in the bottle. Sometimes I will go back and open up a bottle just to recount it."

"Here is your new prescription, Jeremy."

Obsessive-compulsive disorder is indeed a component of the bipolar spectrum and, therefore, a component of chronic pain. I will return to this subject in a later chapter, but I did want to share Jeremy's experience with you.

Just a short while later, I took a phone call from him. He told me his lawyer wanted him off of the Methadone. I scheduled an appointment.

He was obviously upset. He was wringing his hands together, and he told me through tears that the court date for his divorce was coming up, and that his lawyer had advised him that he must come off the Methadone if he had any hope of obtaining shared custody of his child.

"Jeremy, this comes up a lot. I have seen it a bunch of ways. I have seen it in divorces, custody battles, inheritances, lost jobs, the whole nine yards. It is the idea that people taking opiates are addicted and, therefore, impaired and irresponsible. I don't want you off the Methadone. You need it, and need it badly. It is controlling your disease. Could I simply send your lawyer a letter stating that you are on Methadone for the treatment of pain?" I wouldn't dare mention bipolarity—what would that do for Jeremy's chances? "Would that not be sufficient?"

"No," he said. "My lawyer tells me that this judge believes that everyone taking Methadone is a heroin addict. I think somebody in his family, maybe it was his son, had trouble with drugs and was on Methadone. I have got to come off of it. My lawyer tells me there is nothing else I can do. A letter will do no good at all. I have to be off Methadone when I go to court."

"Okay, Jeremy, what I am going to do is increase the dose of your Oxycodone, and we are going to do a taper on your Methadone. You are not taking a big dose, and I think you ought to be able to come off of it pretty well, maybe over the course of just a few days. So reduce it by a half a pill a day. I think we can cover your pain and maybe your nervousness and all the rest with more Oxycodone."

Jeremy got by with the extra Oxycodone. He was able to come off Methadone without any withdrawal. Gradually, however, his depression, anxiety, restlessness and thought scatter reappeared. I increased yet again his Oxycodone, and although he hardly prospered, he was still able to work at the body shop. When the divorce proceedings were finally concluded and Jeremy received with his wife divided custody of their child, he was able to resume, mercifully, his Methadone. He was once again mood stabilized and pain diminished but at the price of taking more opiate than when he entered divorce court.

So all is more or less well. My patient is doing satisfactorily, but I do harbor resentment that a divorce court judge, who really knows very little about Methadone or opiate therapy, should dictate what I, who know quite a lot about it, should do in the care of my patient. I can live with it, but I don't like it. I don't like the stigma that is attached to those who take opiates in general, and Methadone in particular. And I don't like a legal system that presumes that those taking opiates are guilty until proven innocent.

A nearby manufacturing company mandated that all its employees submit to urine drug testing. All those who tested positive for opiates, even legitimately prescribed (the vast majority), were discharged because of their potential impairment and threat to workplace safety. A class action lawsuit was filed. My name as a pain doctor and the prescribing physician for some of the employees appeared in several depositions.

I took a call from a *New York Times* reporter. I told her that, in my opinion, the firings were unjust. I also told her that I was glad there was a lawsuit to address, at a societal level, how we handle people who are obliged by illness to take opiates for pain. I simmered in slow outrage that night, and the next morning called her back to tell her I had more things to say. She was happy to hear me out. I told her that people taking opiates were doing so for a disease that impairs. Chronic pain impairs memory, attention, mood, sleep, disposition, and even motor skills, and these impairments can be diminished, sometimes greatly, by opiate therapy. I emphasized that those taking opiates are often better and safer workers than they would be without the drugs. She thanked me for my remarks and told me that the president of the American Pain Society had told her the very same thing. Her article appeared on the front page of the *New York Times* October 25, 2010. It is archived on the *Times* Web site and presents a balanced view of a very important societal issue.

CHAPTER 5

The Spectrum

A clinical state of persistent sadness and inability to experience pleasure has been recognized since antiquity and identified as *melancholia*. It means, quite literally, black bile, a derivative of the ancients' belief that disease was a product of some abnormality of the body's *humors* or liquids. Not until the twentieth century was melancholia replaced by our current terminology, (major) depression.

It was in the late nineteenth century that physicians began to observe a very curious phenomenon in some of their patients with melancholia. This was the sudden appearance of a dramatic change in mood and behavior characterized by hyperactivity and elation. It was the polar opposite of melancholia. This state was identified as *mania*, from the Greek, "madness." Thus was born manic-depressive disorder.

In our current lexicon, we recognize major or unipolar (for obvious reason) depression and a lesser variant that is identified as *dysthymia* (disordered mood). We now identify manic-depressive disorder as bipolar disorder and divide it into two major groups, Bipolar I and II. Bipolar I is the classic bipolarity characterized by the presence of mania, usually recurrent, of at least a week's duration. Bipolar II is a lesser expression of the disorder with the amplitude of mood swings being diminished and of shorter duration. Thus, the term *hypomania* (less than mania). The distinction between the two forms of bipolarity can be stated succinctly. A Bipolar I has great difficulty functioning as a competitive member of society. A Bipolar II can function and often very well. Subject to intervals of depression to be sure, he or she nonetheless possesses the bipolar attributes of high energy and quickness in thought and wit.

There is another disorder characterized by mood shifts, and it is recognized as *cyclothymia* (cycling mood). Many physicians, certainly myself included, recognize cyclothymia as "*soft*" bipolarity. It is often a *subclinical* disease, meaning the person does not know they are sick—only that they are somewhat sad, irritable, and subject to mood shifts and attacks of anger with the least provocation (road rage is an example). I will write a lot about these people in this book because it is the appearance of pain, not their emotional symptoms, that drive them to see the doctor.

The subdivision of mood disorders into several subtypes is a helpful diagnostic tool, but the distinctions are rather unimportant so far as therapy is concerned. Those drugs that are used to treat Bipolar I are also used to treat Bipolar II and soft bipolarity. And those drugs that are used to treat major depression are also used for dysthymia. Moreover, those drugs that are used for the treatment of depression are often used in the treatment of bipolar disorder and vice versa. Indeed, psychiatrists and primary care physicians are increasingly employing mood stabilizers for the treatment of major depression, often with great benefit. This raises an important issue, one that is in the back of the minds of many physicians. How many depressives are indeed bipolars who have not been manic—yet? Maybe it is all one disease.

Now let's talk about mania. It is an altered emotional and behavioral state characterized in the classic example by elevated mood but probably more commonly by anxiety, irritability, thought racing, and sleeplessness. A few of the people I write about in this book describe mania as a "phenomenal" or "euphoric" experience—one that gives great pleasure. But part of that pleasure is the exhibition of recklessness and disinhibition that lead to self-destructive behaviors, be these social, financial, or sexual. Such behaviors are understandably destructive to relationships, and multiple marriages and divorces are not uncommon in the bipolar. I will offer many examples of manic interludes in this book, and you will see that they come in great variety.

Perhaps surprisingly to you, depression and mania may occur simultaneously, a *mixed* state. In its most vivid expression it creates an irritable, angry, energized person who is empowered to act upon his worst thoughts, thus suicidality and homicidality. I believe that most bipolars in pain are in a sort of mixed state in which they are chronically depressed, painful, irritable, sleep-deprived, fatigued, inattentive, forgetful, and often dream ridden. Their mania is an occasional feeling, for a day or two, of being "normal." Clearly, there are instances in which pain and depression, or perhaps better a mixed state, occur cyclically. This may be throughout the day, the month (female bipolars often have a real problem during their menstrual period), or the year. It is this cyclicity of pain and depression that can be a very good clue to bipolarity, and I will offer several examples.

The concept of the bipolar spectrum, also known as the *mood disorder spectrum* or *affective disorder spectrum* (the distinction is unimportant—*spectrum* is the operative word) has vastly increased the breadth of the disease. Just how many mental illnesses it encompasses depends on which psychiatrist you talk to. In this book I will explore, always in relationship to chronic pain, attention deficit disorder (ADD), obsessive-compulsive disorder (OCD), narcolepsy, post-traumatic stress disorder (PTSD), and multiple personality disorder (MPD). The latter two, I remind you, are often the sequelae of childhood sexual abuse. Thus, a link between that experience and bipolar disorder.

Attention deficit disorder has many features in common with bipolarity. It is characterized by inattentiveness, distractibility, mind racing, impulse, hyperactivity, and restlessness—all features of bipolar mania. (I will no longer make a distinction between mania and hypomania. The former will refer to both.) In the classic sense, it should be quite easy to distinguish between ADD and bipolarity. The former usually appears in youth and the latter in adulthood. Another distinction is that the symptoms of ADD are persistent and those of bipolar mania intermittent. However, if both are within the compass of the bipolar spectrum, why is there really a need to make a distinction?

A word now about *attention deficit hyperactivity disorder* (ADHD). That, indeed, is a disorder of childhood. Although adult attention deficiency is not conventionally thought to be associated with hyperactivity, I do see periodic hyperactivity, behavioral as well as mental, in some of my patients with ADD, and I will share these cases with you in the course of this book. I ask as you read them that you reflect on whether what I am describing is adult attention deficit hyperactivity disorder or bipolar mania. The distinction is not easy of accomplishment at all. But it really doesn't matter. Both can, and often do, respond to the same drugs. Lastly, it is well recognized that many children with ADD or ADHD become adults with bipolar disorder.

After I learned of the bipolar spectrum, I began inquiring about symptoms of inattention and distractibility in my patients. I have been somewhat surprised at the frequency of the affirmative response and also by just how disabling these symptoms can be. My patients react to my queries with great emotion, sometimes crying and expressing frustration over their inability to think. They tell me that they simply can't remember as they should, that they have to write reminder notes to themselves, that they cannot complete tasks, and that they can no longer read books because they cannot comprehend and retain the material.

Obsessive-compulsive disorder is characterized by a persistently intrusive and commanding, often fearful, thought (the obsession) causing the victim to engage in physical acts (compulsions) that protect from the obsession and diminish the anxiety that attends it. Thus, the well-known example of the obsessive and fearful thought that the hands are dirty and covered with germs leads to the physical act of washing the hands throughout the day. OCD can hardly be mistaken for bipolarity although the bipolar may well be subject to mind racing and forced or obsessive thought.

Some of my patients with OCD come to me already on treatment, usually with an SSRI. In most, however, the disorder is, to employ that word again, subclinical. They don't recognize their symptoms as a disease. Rather, they are just a part of their being, and only a few have directed their doctor's attention to them. They almost never do with me. I have to search for it, but I find it frequently. The predominant symptom is obsessive striving for cleanliness and organization within the household or workplace. A common feature is repetitive mental acts such as talking to oneself throughout the day, expressing repetitively the same idea. Another feature is the act of counting—reciting numbers sequentially and ending on one that does not give anxiety. A kindred feature is the need to touch objects when one enters a new environment—a form of counting perhaps. These repetitive acts are, to offer a generalization, anxiety diminishing, and anxiety is common in OCD (and ADD). The two diseases would appear to be quite different. One is a disease of too many, and undisciplined, thoughts, and the other is a disease of a single commanding, intrusive thought. And yet the product of these different forms of thinking can be quite similar—distractibility, inattention, and difficulty reading books.

Narcolepsy, as most know, is a disease characterized by repetitive sleep attacks throughout the day. Another feature is sudden loss of muscle tone causing the victim to fall. This phenomenon is known as *cataplexy*. It is often precipitated by startle or emotional acts such as laughing or crying. It is painless, and there is no alteration of consciousness as there is in a faint. Another feature of narcolepsy, which to my mind is the most defining, is the presence of vivid, threatening dreams. The victim sometimes awakens from them briefly paralyzed and mute, a phenomenon known as *sleep paralysis*. The dreams are quite real to the victims, and they awake highly charged emotionally with feelings of fear, anxiety, or anger. It often takes a while to realize that the dream is not real. These dreams are identified as *hypnagogic* or *hypnopompic hallucinations*. The words, hypnagogic and hypnopompic, have similar meaning. Both refer to the twilight state between wakefulness and sleep—hypnagogic on entering sleep from wakefulness and hypnopompic on entering wakefulness from sleep.

I have already given you examples of people with chronic pain who suffer from very vivid dreams. The incidence of that complaint in those in pain is extraordinarily high. An interesting aside—many bipolars offer a history of night terrors when they were young.

The phenomenon of cataplexy, which I formerly thought was rare, is probably not uncommon in those in pain. It is difficult to make the diagnosis with certainty unless the physician actually witnesses an attack. Many things other than cataplexy can make those in pain fall. As examples, a person with a badly damaged spine will fall occasionally. A person with numb feet from peripheral neuropathy is also subject to falls. I will never let a major clinical decision be made on the basis of whether or not my patient suffers cataplexy because the diagnosis is so often unsure, but I will accept a suggestive history as a clue. A feature among those in pain that I have only begun to explore recently is the rather common complaint of "clumsiness." Those in pain not only fall; they drop things repetitively and unaccountably so. I do wonder if clumsiness and dropping things might be due to a sudden and limited loss of muscle tone, which is perhaps some variant of cataplexy.

Many of those in pain suffer from very vivid dreams with only the softest suggestion of other features of narcolepsy. I consider this another subclinical disorder. Victims believe the dreams, sometimes very terrible dreams, are simply inherent to their nature. They don't recognize them as symptoms of a disease. I do. The presence of these dreams allows me to make at least a tentative diagnosis of narcolepsy. Tentative enough, that is, to invite treatment for that disorder. Remarkably, when I treat the dream-afflicted patient with a stimulant, the pain often goes away. Even more remarkable, when I treat the pain with an opiate, the dreams go away. And this same kind of effect, I see in patients with ADD and OCD. The spectrum again. There is a link; there is a connection between all these disorders and the symptoms they generate.

Post-traumatic stress disorder is a well-recognized product of physical or emotional trauma. It is characterized by anxiety and depression and particularly the reliving of the event, often in response to some trigger that provokes its recollection. In wakefulness, the recreation of the event is known as a *flashback*. The same thing occurs during sleep with the recreation occurring in horrific dreams. The incidence of PTSD, often acquired by sexual trauma, in those in pain, many of whom are also bipolar, is extremely high. Sad but interesting that those in pain so often suffer from both narcoleptic nightmares and post-traumatic nightmares. No wonder so many of them dread the coming of the night.

Post-traumatic stress disorder is not an easy disease to treat. We conventionally employ antidepressants and anxiolytics, and although we might be able to control some of the anxiety and depression that attend the disease, it is quite difficult, with pharmacy, to make the flashbacks go away. Perhaps one of the most remarkable observations that I have made is that flashbacks and bad dreams can be ameliorated, sometimes totally inhibited, in people who suffer from pain and the bipolar spectrum by the administration of drugs such as opiates and stimulants. I have already given an example, and there will be many more.

Multiple personality disorder, also known as *dissociative identity disorder*, describes the existence within a single person of two or more totally different personalities. These personalities are each unique with their own chronological age, speech, mannerisms, and behavior. The disorder often stems from childhood trauma, particularly sexual abuse, and among the personalities there is, almost invariably, one of a child of the age when sexual trauma was experienced. Another is often a commanding, angry, shall we say more protective, personality. The technical word for these shifts between personalities is *dissociation*, an entry into a new state of being (the same word can be applied to bipolarity, thus a manic dissociation into a new state of being). A near universal attribute of multiple personality disorder is that after the dissociation, the victim has no memory of the experience. Thus, many people with MPD have gaps, sometimes very large gaps, in their memory. A link between multiple personality disorder and bipolar disorder would, on the face of it, appear highly unlikely. That is what I thought until I cured multiple personality disorder in two bipolars by the administration of opiates. That, I assure you, is just about the most astonishing thing I have ever seen.

A word now about the *metabolic syndrome*, a disease almost epidemic in our society. It is the comorbidity of obesity, hypertension, and diabetes.

These three diseases are now thought to be biochemically linked, perhaps not unlike the linkage we find in the bipolar spectrum. Thus, several seemingly unrelated disorders derive from a common cause. So, what does the metabolic syndrome have to do with the bipolar spectrum? Maybe a lot.

Psychiatrists are increasingly looking at the relationship between mental disorders and physical disorders. What could be the relationship between depression and, say, inflammatory diseases such as rheumatoid arthritis? And what is the relationship of bipolarity (and chronic pain) to obesity, hypertension, and diabetes? It is not nearly as far-fetched as you might think. I am beginning to see people in the bipolar spectrum with treatment-resistant hypertension experience control of their blood pressure when drugs such as opiates and even stimulants (which should raise blood pressure) are administered. On a few occasions, I have seen diabetes better controlled under the same scenario. This leaves us with obesity, extremely prevalent in the bipolar and in those in pain. It is no coincidence that several of the people I describe in this book, all bipolars, have undergone gastric bypass surgery. I have already given you an example of a man on opiate therapy who lost much needed weight. This happens quite a lot in the bipolar in pain. It is understandable that the obese bipolar in pain will often lose weight with stimulant therapy. But why they should lose it with opiate therapy is much less certain to me.

Now I want to discuss chronic pain as a part of the bipolar spectrum. An overview is necessary. There are many people who suffer from chronic pain due to arthritis, and there are people with migraine who suffer from recurrent pain. And there are many other examples of chronic pain. Many of these people *do not* suffer from depression nor do they suffer from disordered sleep, appetite, energy, mood, thought, and all the rest. They suffer from chronic pain, *the condition*, and that is quite different from chronic pain, *the disease*, that which is associated almost invariably with psychiatric illness.

It is not my intent to particularly identify or really to pay much regard to the individual painful states because, I believe, they all represent a single core illness, one closely aligned with the bipolar spectrum. I will, however, mention a few common ones. Fibromyalgia is a disease of chronic muscular pain. It does, in the minds of some rheumatologists, have defining features, but other rheumatologists question its very existence. Migraines have been around forever, and of the painful states, it has the most defining behavior with periodic headache, often unilateral (one-sided), attended by visual effects such as blurring or *scintillations* (sparkles) in the visual field and *photosonophobia*, which means painful sensitivity to light and sound. Remarkably, of all of the states of pain, migraine is the one most often relieved by sleep. The so-called tension headache, now better identified as chronic daily headache or *transformed migraine*, is an incessant head pain that has none of the defining features of migraine. The term, transformed migraine, refers to the fact that most people with chronic headaches have a history of migraine, which is transformed into another form of pain. This transformation usually occurs under the provocation of some emotional or physical trauma, one that induces depression, and I will offer examples in this book. The *failed back* identifies ongoing pain after back surgery. A word now about back surgery because it is will be referenced so much in this book. A disc (the cushion between the vertebrae) ruptures and presses upon a nerve producing pain down the leg (sciatica). This ruptured disc can be removed surgically, but if vertebral alignment is displaced by ruptured discs or arthritis, a larger operation, the fusion of the vertebrae together, is required. Thus, many people in this book will have experienced either a *cervical* (neck) fusion or a *lumbar* (low back) fusion. Many, in the course of their care, are subjected to a form of therapy that consists of injections of cortisone near the nerves exiting the spine. This is known as the *epidural steroid injection*. It is a conservative and relatively harmless form of therapy, and it occasionally works.

I need to emphasize that none of the individual painful states really fit into a box. They overlap simultaneously or sequentially in time. Thus, the person with migraine often develops fibromyalgia. The failed back often becomes comorbid with fibromyalgia, and fibromyalgia comorbid with nearly everything.

The different painful states have many features in common. Most lack defining pathology that we can image by X-ray, CAT scan, or MRI. They all lack defining blood or urine tests. Many of them represent a *failure to recover* from illness or injury. Thus, the muscular sprain or overuse injury does not go away but evolves into fibromyalgia. The chronic back pain, accountable on the basis of a ruptured disc, does not go away when the disc is surgically removed. Thus, the failed back. The periodic migraine becomes incessant, transformed into chronic headache. And the list goes on.

Lastly, the various states of chronic pain almost always have a common symptomology. I will briefly review this and in doing so point out the similarities between chronic pain and the bipolar spectrum.

Sleep in those in pain is disordered in many ways. Pain often worsens at night. It is frequently disturbed by mind racing (OCD, ADD, and bipolarity). Certain tremors, notably restless legs and periodic jerking movements, are common as is, strangely, nocturia—frequent voidings through the night. Sleep is interrupted by vivid dreams, often threatening (narcolepsy, PTSD).

Appetite is disordered. It is diminished in some with weight loss but more commonly increased with weight gain and obesity (bipolarity, metabolic syndrome).

Those in pain suffer from a want of energy. Their sleep is nonrestorative, and they experience fatigue and daytime sleepiness (narcolepsy).

Mood is disordered, usually with depression but also with irritability, anger, anxiety, and restless, usually purposeless, hyperactivity (bipolarity, ADD) but sometimes with purposeful but inefficient and useless hyperactivity (OCD).

Thought is disordered with thought-scatter and mind-racing (bipolarity, ADD), unwanted and obsessive thought, and sometimes an inability to think about anything other than the pain (OCD).

Memory and mental focus are impaired in those in pain with distractibility, forgetfulness, memory loss, and difficulty with comprehension (ADD, OCD, and MPD).

Motor skills are impaired, and the painful, with great frequency, describe themselves as "clumsy," subject to tripping and falling and dropping things (? cataplexy).

To summarize, the vastness of the bipolar spectrum encompasses the vastness of chronic pain. Whether we say it all represents a single illness or a continuum is really, to my mind, a moot point because in this book I will demonstrate time and time again the benefits of appropriate pharmacy with those benefits extending across all of the diagnostic categories.

CHAPTER 6

Dreams

I have always enjoyed the initial patient interview. I like connecting the dots, exploring the relationships between my patients' symptoms and the stories of their lives. With an appreciation now of the bipolar spectrum and the enormous breadth of the disease, there are a lot more dots. Some of them, which I previously considered trivial and unimportant, have become highly relevant and have led me to several ideas regarding treatment. Such is the case with dreams, a near universal human experience but a very malevolent one in the bipolar in pain.

Roger was thirty-eight years old, the father of two and, until his injury, a heavy equipment mechanic. He hurt his back at work some two years before coming to me and was found to have a ruptured disc. Surgery was performed, but his improvement was brief, and a second operation to remove yet another disc was done six months later. It too failed, and postoperatively, he developed loss of sensation in the genital and rectal areas. His sexual activity was impaired, and he could tell he needed to have a bowel movement only by sudden increase in pain in his back. His orthopedist told him that if his pain did not abate, he would need a lumbar fusion. That is when he came to me.

He acknowledged that he was quite sleepless since his pain appeared, and it often worsened at night. He was anxious and found himself worrying a lot, particularly when he tried to go to sleep. I continued my interrogations and asked if he was depressed. He responded, as my patients so often do, by saying, "I don't know."

He was. He described intervals of feeling quite well, even empowered, with these feelings lasting a day or so. The rest of the time, he said, "I am just taking up space." Mental focus and memory were impaired. He was finding himself becoming very distracted and forgetful, and for the first time in his life, he had to write notes to himself to remind him of certain tasks to be done. He told me he had gained weight due to his inactivity, and he acknowledged a certain food craving, that for cabbage, heavily salted. He would lust for that foodstuff for days at a time.

I reflected on what he had told me. He was sleepless, depressed, mood-shifting, inattentive, and had failed two lumbar spine operations. There remained another line of inquiry.

"Roger, do you dream at night?"

He hesitated then looked at me rather quizzically and said, "Yes, I've had bad dreams all my life. Why in the world did you ask me that question?"

"It may be important. Tell me about them. Are they threatening? Do you awaken from them emotional, frightened, anxious, or angry?"

"Yes! They are very threatening. I hate them. When I awaken from them, I am almost always crying and frightened."

"What do you dream about?"

"Demons and things like that."

"Supernatural things?"

"Yes."

"Do you wake up from them with a sense that you are paralyzed, that you can't speak or move?"

"Yes, that happens almost every time. It used to scare me, but I am used to it now. It goes away in just a few moments, but for a while, I am totally paralyzed."

"Do you get sleepy during the day? Do you ever nod off or have to struggle to stay awake during the day?"

"Yes, that happens a lot. I nod off for no reason."

"How long does the sleep last?"

"Just a few minutes."

"And when it is over, how do you feel?"

"Really pretty good. It seems to refresh me."

"Roger, let me ask you a strange question. Do you ever have spells where your legs give out with you for no reason, where you fall down?"

"Yes, but they don't happen very often. Sometimes I just find myself on the floor not knowing how I got there."

"Is it a painful experience, or do you black out?"

"No, I've had them even before I had the back pain."

"Do you find that you are clumsy, that you drop things?"

"Yes, but that is just since the pain struck me. I drop things a lot. I have broken lots of coffee cups."

My patient was narcoleptic, heretofore unsuspected and undiagnosed. There are many reasons for this, but one of them begins with Roger. He had never directed his doctor's attention to these symptoms, I am sure because he did not view them as an illness but rather just as a part of his life. His narcolepsy was, thus, a subclinical illness. It was not until he had pain, two years of it, that his underlying narcolepsy and bipolar spectrum was recognized.

I prescribed the stimulant, Ritalin, and the anxiolytic and anticonvulsant, Klonopin. I will remind the reader that both of these drugs are held in low esteem by many practitioners because of the capacity for abuse and addiction, and in the case of Klonopin, sedation and loss of balance. This, I suggest, is an example of weighing the potential harm from a drug against the probability of benefit. This is a theme that will recur throughout this book as I tell the stories of those in pain.

When I saw him next, he told me that he was feeling better. His sleep was more restorative, but he was continuing to have nod-off attacks during the day, and his primary care doctor had scheduled him for a sleep study. I told him to increase the dose of the medicines and also that I would be most interested in the findings from the sleep study.

Polysomnography is a measurement, during sleep, of a variety of body functions including brainwave activity, cardiac and respiratory function, and eye and limb movement. Assembled together, this data allows the physician to make a diagnosis of one of several different sleep disorders. Much the most common is *sleep apnea*, a disorder in which breathing is impaired to the point of temporary cessation during sleep. That was Roger's diagnosis.

A month later Roger was much improved. He no longer got sleepy during the day, his energy and mental focus were restored, and he found that he wanted to do more things rather than just take up space. His bad dreams had gone away altogether, and he told me that although he still had pain, it didn't "bother" him as much. Roger continued to do well as I gradually increased his Ritalin dosage. I scheduled his return visits out to every three months. During that interim, I received a letter from his referring orthopedist. It recounted in detail his history of prior surgeries for disc disease and the recent reappearance of severe back pain radiating to his legs. He had developed weakness in his left leg and had difficulty walking. His imaging studies showed another disc ruptured and massively so at that.

Moreover, the vertebra was slipping backward. Spinal stability was being lost. He required another operation—a lumbar fusion.

I saw Roger barely a month from that operation. He told me he was doing "tolerably well" with recovery from his leg weakness and pain. He continued to extol the Ritalin and Klonopin, drugs that had arrested his dreams, his inattention and forgetfulness, his daytime sleepiness, and his depression. He was no longer mood-shifting, he told me, and his lust for cabbage was almost totally abated.

I have had to add Hydrocodone to control Roger's pain, but in the main he is doing well. Some people are destined for back trouble, and he is certainly one of them. Where does the bipolar spectrum fit in? One would hardly suggest that his bipolarity had anything to do with his ruptured discs, but could it not have something to do with his perception of pain?

Before leaving Roger, we need to reflect on the fact that his sleep study, currently the gold standard for diagnosing sleep disorders, revealed no evidence of narcolepsy. Admittedly, that diagnosis sometimes requires a special derivation of the sleep study known as the *sleep latency test*, and that was not performed, presumably because his physicians felt they had a secure diagnosis, that of sleep apnea. This is often the case. Daytime somnolence is quite common in those who suffer from chronic pain, and many of my patients have had sleep studies performed. Almost never have they revealed narcolepsy. Why is this? I really don't know, but before the sleep study was developed as a diagnostic tool in the 1970s, we made the diagnosis of narcolepsy solely on the medical history. The description of realistic, threatening dreams, sleep paralysis, daytime sleepiness, and the falling spells of cataplexy, or at least some of those, was sufficient to make a diagnosis of narcolepsy. I suppose my diagnosis was correct for stimulant therapy, highly appropriate for narcolepsy, and rather inappropriate for sleep apnea corrected his disordered sleep and with it mood shifting, inattentiveness, depression, and to some extent, pain. These were all, I am sure you have noticed, expressions of the bipolar spectrum.

Lastly, what did the craving for heavily salted cabbage really mean? It came on when he became painful, and it went away when I gave him Klonopin and Ritalin. I will return to the interesting subject of such cravings in those in pain in a later chapter.

Cathy was thirty years old when she came to see me. She was married and working regularly. Her first child was born just six months before. Her headaches began about age twenty, and they were typical migraines. They occurred predominantly over the right side of her head, and they were throbbing in character with photosonophobia. Their duration was of up to twenty-four hours. They were quite frequent, occurring almost daily and often awakening her from her sleep in the morning. She probably inherited the disease because both parents were migraine sufferers. She consulted a neurologist and was treated with anticonvulsants—first Depakote, which was ineffective and produced weight gain, and then Neurontin, also ineffective and sedating. Over the course of a few years she was prescribed several different drugs of the triptan class. These can be very effective in arresting a migraine attack, but she had bad luck with them. One of them, Maxalt, gave her heart palpitations. She did report that she was subject to severe headaches during her menstrual period. Other triggers were heat and exercise. She denied depression or anxiety.

Cathy seemed to me to be an emotionally healthy and stable person cursed with migraines that had, at least thus far, not responded to appropriate therapy. I elected to try yet another anticonvulsant, that known as Keppra. It was too sedating, so I tried Topamax. Its side effect was a sensation of tingling in the face and hands, but she was willing to tolerate that because it was the first drug that had ever given her any relief from her headaches. She did well for a year and a half and then came to me complaining, for the first time, of anxiety and depression. Her headaches, nonetheless, remained in good control. I prescribed Cymbalta, but she tolerated it very poorly. I changed to Paxil with the addition of the anxiolytic, Xanax. She did rather well on that combination for a matter of several months and then experienced a severe migraine, one of the worst ever, causing her to go to the emergency room. After that, depression and anxiety recurred full force.

It was time for reappraisal. My patient, nearly two and half years under my care, was back to square one. Armed now with knowledge of the bipolar spectrum and its relation to pain in general and migraines in particular, I inquired if she suffered vivid dreams. She acknowledged that she did, but she denied experiencing sleep paralysis or anything resembling cataplexy. She did volunteer, however, that she was suffering sleep attacks during the day, sometimes falling asleep for as long as twenty minutes. She denied mood shifts except, she told me, that when she had a migraine she felt intensely angry, an emotion she had not experienced with her headaches until recently. And yes, she said, she was having trouble with distractibility and an inability to multitask. She was moving from one task to another without completing any of them. Moreover she had become very sleep-disturbed.

I felt my patient in pain was evolving, as those with pain often do, into the bipolar spectrum. What to do? Conventional mood stabilizer therapy was not attractive to me because she had already failed Depakote, Neurontin, Keppra, and now, Topamax. All were given for her migraines, but all can be effective mood stabilizers. I wanted to jump in with psychostimulant therapy, but at that time I was not as convinced of its safety in the bipolar with migraines as I am now. So I elected to go with Klonopin. It is helpful for sleep, and some people with migraine and bipolarity do quite well with the drug. I wrote a prescription for it, but I hedged my bet by giving her a second prescription—that for Adderall. I told her to try the Klonopin first and to contact me in a couple of weeks regarding her progress. If she was not better, she could get the Adderall prescription filled.

She reported almost complete recovery with the Klonopin. Her anxiety and depression had diminished, and her headaches had nearly gone away. At that juncture she was taking Topamax, Klonopin, Xanax, and Paxil. She was doing so well that I scheduled her return visit for six months. There was no need for the Adderall. I told her to discard the prescription.

She got about a year out of the Klonopin and other medications, and then she relapsed full force with return of daytime nod-offs, threatening dreams, anxiety, and migraine. Once again, I wrote a prescription for Adderall up to 20 mg daily. The effect was almost immediate with her recovery being far more complete than it had been with the Topamax or Klonopin. Along the way I have increased the dosage, and for the first time in fifteen years, five of them under my care, she has achieved near total relief from migraine and, with it, recovery from depression, nightmares, daytime sleepiness, inattention, and distractibility.

I believe Cathy falls into the bipolar spectrum, and I know I have taken great liberties with the diagnostic tables, as I so often do. I did not feel the need to obtain a sleep study to diagnose narcolepsy. And I will admit her symptoms of that disease were somewhat limited. I would have liked more, and that was the reason I deferred stimulant therapy, at least initially, in favor of Klonopin. Be advised that no psychiatrist would make a diagnosis of bipolarity in this woman, but I did and by doing so, I helped her. All my experience tells me that she will continue to do well on her current therapy.

A point of interest is that Cathy's disease evolved over time, and this often happens. At onset she had typical migraine. It was, however, migraine unresponsive to conventional therapy, and this, I believe, is a clue to underlying bipolarity. Years into her illness she began to develop depression and anxiety, and then distractibility and inattention, vivid dreams, daytime sleep attacks, and migraine-induced anger. This kind of scenario, this evolution over time, will be examples repeatedly in this book.

Cathy's migraine was the first symptom of her bipolar spectrum, at least the first that took her to a doctor. In others to be described in this book, pain is a late symptom of bipolarity. So, the chicken and the egg—which comes first? We can avoid that conundrum by accepting that bipolarity is inherent in many, perhaps most of us, and will express itself in different ways at different times in our lives.

Linda, age thirty-nine, came to me in 1997. She was referred by her orthopedist regarding her chronic back pain. Several years before, she felt a sudden pop in her back with pain radiating down the right leg. She came to surgery for a ruptured lumbar disc and did quite well—for three years. And then her pain recurred just as before. A second operation was performed, this time without benefit, and she was given the low-order opiate, Darvocet, which gave some relief, but she had become progressively sleepless and depressed. Perhaps with good reason. Her mother was diagnosed with cancer about the time of her second operation, and although the family was given a good prognosis, mother deteriorated rapidly and died within three months.

Linda told me that she suffered restless legs and, according to her husband, "jerkings" at night. These were almost certainly a nocturnal tremor known as *periodic limb movement,* a sort of flailing of the extremities that occurs during sleep. It is not uncommon—particularly so in those who suffer from chronic pain. Linda also told me that for the past year or so she had had a problem with migraines, but it was fairly well controlled with Propranolol and Verapamil. These drugs are used to treat high blood pressure, but they are also sometimes effective in the prevention of migraines. I put migraines on the back burner and initiated treatment with Klonopin and Imipramine, my usual start-ups at that time and often even now. She responded rather well. Her back pain was diminished. Her sleep was restored, and her tremors diminished.

I was pleased with what had been achieved. Linda was a long way from well, but she was better, and with the aid of Darvocet, she was getting by well enough to home school her two children. It went along well for many years. She was functioning at a high level, and although she continued to experience occasional intervals of depression, I made no major changes in her therapy. I saw her only every six months, and I enjoyed her visits for she is a charming and intelligent woman. She occasionally offered the complaint, however, that her migraines were still a bother. She had discontinued the Propranolol and Verapamil, thinking them ineffective. I prescribed Maxalt, and she reported a good response with near immediate cessation of migraine. Unfortunately, she had to take it at great frequency, something on the order of one a day, and that is a lot.

The triptans are blood vessel constrictors with the capacity to cause heart attacks and strokes. Uncommon probably, but still a threat. It was time to move into *prophylactic* therapy, the administration of a drug to prevent migraine rather than to treat it after it occurs. I choose Topamax, a drug with a good track record for preventing migraine, and she found it quite effective. It was, however, sedating, and this effect is well known—so much so that the drug is identified in the vernacular as Dopamax. I discarded it in favor of a kindred drug, Keppra. The same effect—sleepiness and sedation. Next Lamictal, with the same outcome—prevention of migraine but ongoing sleepiness.

Time to rethink the issue. Linda and I were now in 2007, a decade from when I first saw her, totally unaware of the bipolar spectrum then but very much aware now.

"Linda, do you dream?"

"How did you know that? I have had crazy dreams all my life. They do bother me, but I never thought I could do anything about it."

"Do you awaken from these dreams emotional?"

"Yes, very emotional. The dreams are real to me, and they are very threatening. I am fearful when I awake."

"Do you ever awaken and feel that you are paralyzed, that you can't move?"

"No, but I often dream that I am paralyzed, and when I dream that, I don't know whether it is real or not. It seems real to me."

"Do you have falling spells? Are there times when your legs give out with you? Do you suddenly drop things without cause?"

"Dr. Cochran, you are beginning to scare me. Yes, it happens a lot. What does it mean?"

"I'll get to that later, but this business of being sleepy throughout the day, we had blamed that on the medicines you are taking. I wonder if it could be something else? Is that possible?"

"Yes, I've had a problem with getting sleepy during the day for a long time. Sometimes when I am driving, I have to pull over to the side of the road and take a nap."

"Linda, I believe you have narcolepsy, and that offers us a real clue. I am prescribing the drug, Ritalin. Hopefully, it will arrest your bad dreams and your sleepiness, and if we are lucky, diminish your migraines, and if we are really lucky, relieve your back pain."

"I can't believe that could happen."

"It may, Linda. Keep your fingers crossed."

She told me that when she started the Ritalin, she developed an intense headache. It lasted several hours, and it was followed by what she described as a "halo of pain," a sense of discomfort around her forehead, her temples, and the back of her skull. Nonetheless, she elected to continue. Within a few days her halo of pain disappeared, and she felt a sense of energy, purpose, and well-being that she had not known for a long time. She told me, excitedly, that relatives in Maryland told her how much better she sounded on the phone, so much more confident and positive. Her husband has seen it also. Formerly using thirty-six Maxalt tablets a month, she was down to one or two. The bad dreams had gone away and her daytime sleepiness also.

I have written before that when the right drug kicks in, everything gets better. Well, almost everything. Linda continued to have back pain although she told me that it was diminished, and that the Ritalin seemed to make the Darvocet work better.

Once again, I had successfully treated a disease that I did not know existed when I first encountered her. I wonder if I had been wiser and knowledgeable of the bipolar spectrum (in her case narcolepsy, migraine, depression, and chronic back pain) and had treated her thirteen years ago at the time of her second operation and her mother's death, could I have relieved not only her migraine but her back pain as well? I wish I knew the answer to that question.

Claudette was fifty when she came to me. Her *affect*, that is, her emotional bearing, caught my eye immediately. She appeared very sad, and she spoke with great hesitation, choosing each word with care. I sensed I was in the presence of despair and hopelessness. Some of it, I was to learn, was familial for both of her parents were severe depressives. A sister was bipolar, and one of her four children also.

Her back pain began in her twenties. It was due to *spondylolisthesis*, a displacement of the vertebral bodies and loss of their normal vertical alignment. By her age thirty, the pain had become excruciating, and a lumbar fusion was performed with benefit. The pain, however, gradually reappeared, and a second operation, a revision of the prior fusion, was performed at age forty-two. Once again she experienced pain relief. However, in but a few months, she began to suffer from a pain of a different sort. It was in her abdomen. She was found to have a cancer of her colon that had metastasized to the liver. It was an unusual tumor known as *carcinoid*. Unlike most colon cancers that arise from the *mucosa* (inner surface) of the intestines, carcinoid originates from nerve cells within the colon. And carcinoid nerve cells do what nerve cells are supposed to do. They release neurotransmitters, including serotonin, the very transmitter that in wellness maintains our mood. Released unrestrained in the bloodstream, however, it causes periodic attacks of flushing of the skin, diarrhea, and occasionally wheezing. Claudette suffered these in abundance until her surgery when the cancer and the diseased portion of her liver were removed. Following this, her symptoms disappeared—for about a year. Then the flushing and diarrhea recurred exactly as before. This was clear evidence that the tumor was still alive some place in her body, but it could not be located by any imaging study. Thus, for the past six years she had an almost daily reminder that her cancer was still within her and would, surely, sooner or later make its location known. On top of this, her back pain recurred as before and her abdominal pain also. No certain cause for either could be identified. She was given Cymbalta for her depression and Oxycodone for her pain and referred to me.

She told me she was somewhat uncomfortable with the Cymbalta although, strangely, it diminished her serotonin-induced diarrhea. Her sleep had been poor for years. She was subject to frequent painful awakenings. Fatigue, she acknowledged, was a major issue also. I wrote her a prescription for Imipramine and Klonopin, and told her that I thought there was hope for recovery. Seemingly unmoved by my remarks, she left looking as sad as when she came.

As I dictated my consultation note, I realized that I had not been able to engage this woman on an emotional level. I found her medical, personal, and family history to be quite remarkable, and her treatment was going to be a challenge, and I certainly welcome that sort of obligation. I remember this quite clearly—I had no sense of commitment on her part, and I had some doubts as to whether she would return to see me again.

My doubts were justified. She did return, but only a year and a half later. I asked her why she had not returned before, and she told me, lamely, that it was because of personal issues, having to take care of her father and such. I then asked her why she *did* come back to me after so long. That question surprised her, and in the first display of spontaneity that I had seen in her, she said, "I think we can tweak it a bit." She then told me that she had tried very hard over the past eighteen months to "get better." She remarked that she actually was better now than when she had seen me over a year before.

If she was better, why did she come back? My patient was lying to herself. She was in denial. Nonetheless, she did return, and I was grateful for the opportunity to treat her. I wrote prescriptions for the same drugs that she had chosen not to take eighteen months before, remarking to myself that only rarely had I ever seen a person so despondent and without hope as Claudette.

"Well, Claudette, it is good to see you again. How are you doing with the new medicine?"

"Maybe a little bit better, just a little bit," she said with something almost approaching a smile.

"Tell me about it."

"Well, the pain in my back and stomach is better, and I don't know how to say this—I just feel maybe more positive."

"That's good. We are moving in the right direction, it is just going to take time," I said, trying to install as much hope as I could.

"There are some problems. I feel sedated on these medicines. I am having a problem with sweats. Could that be due to the drugs?"

"Yes, probably the Imipramine. Let's reduce it a bit. I want to see you back here in three weeks. It does take a while for these drugs to take hold, so it is possible you will continue to improve. Now let's talk about your pain medicine. You have been taking the Oxycodone for several months. Do you feel you need more? I would be happy to prescribe it if you want."

"No, the Oxycodone does help the pain, but I don't like the way it makes me feel. Let's not make any changes right now."

It was three months, not three weeks, before she returned. She offered the same excuses as before. She did tell me that she lost ground. She was crying at the drop of a hat. Some days she said she felt pretty good but mostly she felt down. Her fatigue was overpowering. Her pain was worse, and she volunteered during pain attacks she had great trouble thinking and remembering. It was time to do something different. It was time for a new idea.

"Claudette, are you subject to vivid dreams?"

"Yes, I have had them in the past, dreams that seemed very real, but I don't have them much anymore."

"Do you have a problem with sleepiness or sleep attacks during the daytime?"

"I don't know whether I am sleepy or just exhausted. I do know that I don't sleep at night."

"Claudette, I see from your chart that you had cancelled your appointment for a few weeks ago because of a fall at home. Do you fall a lot?"

"Yes, several times recently I have just suddenly fallen. I don't think it is the pain making me do it. I just suddenly drop to the floor. Do you know what is causing that?"

"Well, maybe. Claudette, I think we touched on this before, but I want to bring it up again. Are you subject to mood shifts now or through your life have you had a problem with that?"

"Yes, maybe a little."

"What is up?"

"Up is normal. Down is depression and pain."

"You told me that when you have a siege of pain you have trouble thinking and you have trouble remembering. Do you become angry when you have pain?"

"No, I don't think so."

As the reader will certainly notice, I was searching hard for clues to the bipolar spectrum. They were there, but barely. Her unexplained falls could have been cataplectic attacks. She probably had suffered hypnagogic hallucinations along the way, but they were infrequent and remote in time. Her mood shifts did not appear extraordinary. I was taken with her volunteering the complaint and mentioning it several times in interview that with her painful spells, she had trouble thinking and remembering. I hear this kind of complaint a lot. Could this be something like ADD? A stretch to be sure. There was no real reason for me to think that this individual was bipolar other than the fact that she had longstanding and treatment-resistant depression, a bipolar attribute, and chronic pain, also a bipolar attribute. Bipolar or not, I had strong grounds for choosing Ritalin. It can be a splendid drug for both unipolar and bipolar depression (although I think it works best in the latter). Moreover, she suffered fatigue, and that certainly merited treatment with a psychostimulant. Ritalin it was.

I was astonished by what I saw on the next visit. She was animated. She was wearing makeup. She looked younger, and she was very pretty.

"Good morning, Claudette, you look so much better."

"That is what my oncologist said. He asked me what medicine I was taking from you, and I told him Ritalin. You will be interested in this. He said, 'RITALIN? How in the world did he think of that?'"

"Thanks for telling me that, Claudette. Looks like I have scored some points with the oncologist."

"Yes, you have, you surely have."

"Tell me what is going on. Obviously the depression is better. How about the rest?"

"The depression is much better. I haven't felt this good in thirty years. My pain doesn't bother me near as much. The Ritalin seems to make the Oxycodone work better if you can believe that."

"I do. Any more falling spells?"

"No, none at all."

"No more thinking or memory problems?"

"Nope."

"And the fatigue—tell me about the fatigue."

"Mostly gone. I have a lot more energy. I feel better when I wake up in the morning because I am sleeping a lot better."

"How long did it take for the Ritalin to start working? How long was it before you knew that something, anything, was different?"

"Within a few hours. All of a sudden the sky was blue again."

"I like that Claudette, I like that a lot."

Claudette has been on Ritalin for over two years and, in the main, has done well. There has been a bump on the road, however, and I want to tell you about it. Claudette and I were informed by her insurer that they would no longer underwrite her Ritalin prescriptions unless she had sleep study confirmation of the diagnosis of narcolepsy or a psychiatric consultation confirming a diagnosis of attention deficit disorder. I had to tell her that the prospect of being diagnosed with either was remote. She would either have to discontinue the Ritalin or pay for it herself. She told me that would be difficult for she didn't have much money.

She came back a month later with a smile on her face and some interesting news. She had told her oncologist about her difficulty obtaining Ritalin. He, the man who had so applauded my choice of the drug, told her the problem was easy of solution. He would write the prescription, and he was sure the insurer would honor it. This was because as an oncologist, treating people with cancer, many of them terminal, he was given great discretion by insurers. His prescriptions were almost never denied. The Ritalin prescription written over his name sailed right through. It is interesting that a cancer doctor can write Ritalin, but a pain doctor cannot. It is a very strange system.

A comment now about the temporal evolution of Claudette's illness. She had, within a matter of a few months, surgery on her back that alleviated back pain and surgery on her abdomen that relieved her abdominal pain. A year of wellness and then nature's announcement, in the form of flushing and diarrhea, that her cancer had returned. It was under this stressor that both her back and abdominal pain reappeared virtually simultaneously. I have written before of pain memories. Past painful experiences can be resurrected by unhappy life events. It happens all the time. It is interesting to me that these reincarnations of pain went away simultaneously and almost totally with Ritalin therapy.

Was Claudette bipolar? I think the evidence dictates yes. It is not because she had a few hypnagogic hallucinations or possibly had cataplexy or had intervals where she couldn't think and remember. It is, in part, because of her strong family history, and we will find this historical feature comes up often in the case studies that follow. It is also in part because she suffered a prolonged and treatment-resistant depression—itself a clue to bipolarity. But the major reason, I believe, was her sudden and total recovery with Ritalin therapy. I see this kind of reaction—when everything gets better, when my patient suddenly looks younger and prettier, and when the sky turns blue again—almost exclusively in bipolars.

Ed was thirty-four, eight years married, expecting his first child, and two years suffering back pain. He had consulted a spine surgeon, and an MRI of the back showed only modest abnormalities. He was given the muscle relaxant, Soma, and Hydrocodone. He found these only moderately helpful. I began my inquiries and learned that his sleep was very disturbed, a problem he had had all his life. With the onset of his pain, he found that the early morning was his most distressful. He would awaken stiff in the back and very painful. During this time, he was aware that he was extremely irritable and fractious. It took him two or three hours to get started on the day, and after that he got by reasonably well—at least until the next morning. He also said, in response to my questions, that he had a very active dream life. He would awaken from dreams anxious and frightened and sometimes briefly paralyzed. He acknowledged depression and worry over his vocational future, for he was subject to flares of pain and irritability causing him to miss an increasing amount of time from work.

"How is your memory, Ed, your mental focus?"

He said, "It is really bad. I am teased at work because I can't seem to finish a job. I will go from one task to another. The same at home. My friends at work and my wife say I have attention deficit disorder."

I prescribed Imipramine and Klonopin. Although my ideas about chronic pain, particularly its relation to the bipolar spectrum, have changed and, with it, my choices of drug therapy, the combination I chose remains, in most cases, a very good start-up program. I could get more creative later if the situation demanded.

Ed got a few good weeks with restoration of sleep and reduction of dreams and even improvement in mental focus. He continued, however, to awaken in the morning with pain and irritability, and after a while his fearful dreams and inattention returned. I chose Methadone.

On his return, he reported some improvement, particularly in his morning pain and irritability. He was actually using less of the Hydrocodone. Over the following weeks, I gradually increased the Methadone dosage up to 60 mg a day. This escalation is usually necessary. There is a pharmacologic threshold, a dose at which everything gets better. Ed told me that his morning irritability and pain had totally disappeared with Methadone, and that his mind wasn't nearly as "scattered." He now was able to follow a schedule and to complete tasks without abandoning them unfinished. His sleep was vastly improved, and he told me his dreams had diminished in frequency, and that they were no longer so threatening to him. When he awoke, he knew it was only a dream and not reality.

Ed exhibited a couple of features very common to those who are in pain. One is the appearance of irritability and often anger with intervals of pain. The other is the strange cyclicity of these attacks, appearing only in the morning. The phenomenon is not rare at all, and I suspect many readers know that. Lastly, he had features, and perhaps only features, of ADD, narcolepsy, and even bipolarity (cyclic irritability). These all went away with Methadone therapy. Please absorb the importance of that. The other people I have told you about in this chapter experienced control of their narcolepsy with psychostimulant therapy. That is what we would expect. But Methadone? I can assure you that Methadone is not conventional therapy for narcolepsy (or for that matter, ADD), but it worked—and quite well. This suggests to me, and I hope to you, that there is a unity, a link between these disorders, and the bipolar spectrum offers us attack from a variety of directions.

Pepper found out about me standing in the checkout line at Walmart. She was talking with her husband about her dreams and her migraines, and one of my patients, similarly afflicted, overheard and introduced herself. She told Pepper about me.

She was thirty-eight years old and the mother of two. She experienced postpartum depression with her first child nine years before. She was treated with Effexor, but it disagreed with her. Gradually, however, she came out of her depression. Then a few years later a catastrophe. Following the birth of her second child, she experienced partial paralysis of her lower extremities, this due to pressure on the nerves of the pelvic floor during delivery. It took her six months to recover, but, she told me, she hadn't been well since. She suffered ongoing depression and, about four years before coming to me, the onset of migraines. It was treatment resistant, this at the hands of a local headache specialist, and also at a faraway headache clinic where she was given the drug, Nardil. It was one of the first antidepressants, and it remains an often effective one, but it carries a risk for interaction with certain foodstuffs such as aged cheese and wine that contain high quantities of tyramine, the metabolic precursor of serotonin. Nardil can also interact with adrenaline-like drugs such as decongestants and also with the opiate, Meperidine. On Nardil and still suffering headaches, she had a bad migraine and went to the emergency room, where she was given a Meperidine injection. In short order, she experienced a hypertensive crisis and epileptic convulsions from which she fortunately recovered (some don't).

She reported mood shifts with periodic distracted hyperactivity and periods of great despondency. She gave a good history of hypnagogic hallucinations almost nightly. She would awaken from these with a sense of anxiety and anger. She also reported that her memory and mental focus were quite poor.

I inquired about her family and childhood. She told me that both of her parents were bipolar. She grew up in a very dysfunctional home. She acknowledged sexual molestation from a neighbor when she was a child. Her medications when I first saw her were Lamictal, Lyrica, Klonopin, Celexa, and Hydrocodone every four hours. In spite of this, she was doing very poorly with headaches sometimes lasting as long as a week. I prescribed Adderall.

On her next visit, she told me that the Adderall had diminished the intensity of her dreams, and that she was sleeping better, but that there had been no change in her headaches. I told her to increase the dose of Adderall, and I wrote a prescription for Methadone at a low dose, 5 mg three times daily. Perhaps I should have waited a bit longer and see what we would get out of Adderall alone, but I have learned that the two drugs together often can be migraine-preventative.

Pepper said she liked the combination. The headaches were diminishing, and she was feeling less depressed and more mentally focused. Then she described a rather bizarre event to me. She kept an appointment with a psychiatrist made by her previous headache doctor. The psychiatrist, reviewing her medications, told her that if she continued to take the Methadone and Adderall, he would refuse to see her. Pepper's protestations, she told me, were to no avail. Even though she told the psychiatrist repeatedly that the medicines were helping her, he refused to attend her.

Oh, well.

Pepper has been under my care now for about six months, and she has continued to improve. I was pleased recently to hear from her husband that for the first time during the two-hour drive to see me Pepper didn't fall asleep. The two had meaningful conversation for the whole trip. Under the sponsorship of Adderall, she began to lose weight, which was much needed, for with her illness, she had become quite obese.

On one of her visits she told me she had found a new psychiatrist she liked very much. He had no problem with my medications at all. He told her that she was bipolar, and he added the mood-stabilizing anticonvulsant Tegretol with benefit. Her new psychiatrist, she told me, said he had read my book and agreed with most of it.

"Thanks for telling me that, Pepper. I know that man, and I respect him. I wouldn't expect him to agree with everything I have written. Most of it is good enough for me."

Pepper is an avid journalist and notekeeper. This type of behavior is not uncommon in those in pain and is probably a reflection of obsessive-compulsive disorder. Regardless, the records can be helpful. On her most recent visit, while on 120 mg of Adderall and 30 mg of Methadone, she showed me her headache calendar. She pointed out that she had gone eighteen days the past month without a headache, which, she said, was "phenomenal."

I wanted to share Pepper's story with you for a couple of reasons. One relates to the simultaneous use of opiates and psychostimulants, a practice that I (and other pain doctors) am employing ever more frequently. The other is that Pepper, unlike the other people in this chapter, did not get well suddenly. Hers was not an abrupt "sky is blue again" recovery. Rather it was slower—one still in evolution. I am confident she will continue to get better, but why most respond quickly and she so slowly I am not sure. It may be that her partial and slow response is because I am not giving her enough medicine yet. There is usually a threshold dosage at which everything finally gets better, and I will return to that subject.

CHAPTER 7

Flashbacks

There is general agreement among psychiatrists that profound emotional trauma carries the potential to disrupt the cerebral infrastructure, that is the neurotransmitter systems (serotonin, noradrenaline, and others) that regulate sleep, appetite, energy, mood, and the perception of pain. Thus, the victim is prey to a host of psychiatric disorders including post-traumatic stress disorder and its companion, chronic pain.

The incidence of sexual abuse in the female population at large is some 25 percent. However, well over 50 percent of my female patients who suffer from pain, and not a few of my males, have suffered sexual abuse, and many more have suffered physical or emotional abuse as well. We know also that some 50 percent of female bipolars, in pain or not, have been sexually abused. While few psychiatrists would suggest that bipolarity is the product of childhood trauma, we do know that the abused child who develops bipolarity will develop it earlier in life and will suffer a higher incidence of suicidality and *rapid cycling*, about which more shortly.

I will suggest that abuse, particularly in childhood, lays the groundwork for the later development of both PTSD and bipolar disorder. The two, in my experience, are so often comorbid with chronic pain that there has to be more than just a chance association. I have already given you an example in the introduction to this book. Recall the abused, bullet-in-the-neck woman who developed first chronic pain, then post-traumatic stress disorder, and then bipolarity. She was cured of all, virtually simultaneously, by the administration of the opiate, Methadone. Does this suggest that by the administration of a drug I was able to cure three different and unrelated diseases, or does it mean that I was able to cure a single disease of which post-traumatic stress disorder, bipolarity, and chronic pain were expressions?

> Dear Dr. Cochran:
>
> This letter is written at the request of Mrs. Peggy Rippy who you will be seeing for the first time. She first came for counseling in 2005 with issues surrounding her son's marriage and issues of conflict with the bride's family and with hostile and rejecting behavior she and her family experience with that family. Most recently she had bladder surgery, and it triggered her issues around sexual abuse she experienced at age 16 with an older man who was her employer at an after school job. She experienced terrific pain and discomfort following the procedure and also became very depressed. She shared for the first time in counseling her experience of the sexual abuse and how she was now recognizing that she had battled depression for many years without understanding the many ramifications of the abuse. She suffers from fibromyalgia and migraine. Reading your recent book, and with the encouragement of her primary care physician and myself, she called for an appointment with you and hopes that you can treat her for her pain and assess and manage her medications for depression. She is a very special person, and I hope you enjoy working with her as much as I do.
>
> Sincerely,
> Michelle Wisdom, LCSW

She was a fifty-five-year-old schoolteacher, attractive and intelligent. I began the interview and learned early on that one of her children was bipolar and a maternal aunt also. Her sexual abuse occurred at age sixteen, and not for forty years did she ever tell anyone about it. At age twenty, away at college, she began to experience migraines, and after a breakup with her boyfriend she suffered an emotional collapse that lead to a six-week stay in a psychiatric hospital. She was diagnosed with bipolarity, and her treatment included, among other drugs, Thorazine and finally Lithium, which did control her mood swings. She ultimately discontinued Lithium and did reasonably well except for periodic flashbacks of her sexual trauma. At age forty-two, she underwent a hysterectomy and within a few days awoke with a sense of "paralysis and an inability to move my body" and intense pain. A diagnosis of fibromyalgia was made. She became sleepless and depressed and subject to more flashbacks. She was given the opiate Hydrocodone and treated with a variety of antidepressants, none of which worked very well. After a year or so, however, her pain and depression gradually remitted. Then after several years of occasional depressive interludes, she underwent bladder surgery. This was extremely painful for her, and in the course of her convalescence her surgeon had a very candid discussion with her about the resumption of sexual activity. This triggered anxiety, depression, mood shifts, and again, flashbacks. She was treated with anxiolytic Ativan, and over the course of the next several years many antidepressants. Unsurprisingly, her fibromyalgia pain reappeared and also worsening migraines. For this disorder she was treated, quite appropriately, with the anticonvulsant, Topamax. It helped a bit at the low dosage of 25 mg a day. If she took more than this, however, her flashbacks increased in frequency and intensity. She reported also that her memory and mental focus were increasingly impaired, and that she was subject to mind-racing and thought-scatter.

My evaluation completed, I concluded that my patient suffered post-traumatic stress disorder, chronic pain in the form of fibromyalgia and migraine, and mood-shifting bipolarity. She was the embodiment of chronic pain and the bipolar spectrum, and she had, quite typically, failed to respond to a variety of antidepressants. I prescribed Ritalin and told her I thought there was a good chance I could help her.

It went well with Peggy, very well. I will let you read it in a note given to me on the occasion of her first return visit.

> Dr. Cochran,
> I had been struggling with MAJOR episodes of mood swings with severe depression and panic attacks. Two hours after taking the Ritalin, I began to notice:
> The tears stopped.
> The depression gradually lifting.
> I began to feel more "level."
> I felt calmer, less anxious.
> I felt less fatigued.
> I could FOCUS, which has been very hard for me to do lately.

My thoughts stopped racing.

Actually after three days on the Ritalin I began to realize I had not felt this "normal" in 13 years—when I was diagnosed with fibromyalgia and had a major depressive/severe pain episode. Throughout my life I have been treated for episodic depression, labeled as postpartum depression, postoperative depression, etc., and was treated with tricyclics, Zoloft, Wellbutrin, Pristiq, and so forth, which did not work. It was amazing that the Ritalin alone connected the missing link in my brain and fixed a broken me. I am now hopeful for the first time in a very long time that my mind is working right.

Having lived with migraines and episodic depression since I was 16 and sexually abused and chronic body pain for the past 13 years, I believe chronic pain DRAINS the soul. It takes so much energy to live with the pain there is just not much left after you do what you have to do. I am fortunate in that I have been able to take advantage of coping programs and develop skills to deal with this, but as I told you, I did get pretty near the end of my rope this year and desperately needed help, so I came to you.

I am now hopeful, since we are headed in the right direction with Ritalin, that the migraines and the insomnia will improve also. The cycling mania/depression is horrible. I would not wish it on anyone.

Sincerely,
Peggy Rippy

I was thrilled with Peggy's progress, but it is never perfect. She told me that the Ritalin was wonderful, but that she would "crash" into depression and sometimes migraine when the effects wore off late in the day. I told her that we could probably prevent that by giving her a sustained release preparation of the drug—one with a longer duration of action. I wrote a prescription for Concerta. As she left she told me that she was going to spend a week on the beach, it being spring vacation. I suggested that she not start the new drug until her return. I don't like the combination of a new drug and a faraway place. I like my patients nearby when I make a change in their therapy, although in this case the change was really quite modest.

Only ten days later, I saw her again. She was much distressed. She handed me another note.

> Wednesday—the Setback
>
> Tuesday—first day back at school after spring break—busy day but nothing unusual. Attended ministry meeting at church that evening—topic was domestic violence including sexual abuse (somewhat unnerving at times). So tired that I slept *eight* hours with no sleep med (incredible). Felt fine upon awakening Wednesday A.M. Took the new medicine instead of Ritalin at 7:00 a.m. Around 9:00 a.m. started feeling BAD, BAD, strange, then felt depressed. Every fifteen minutes or so I would get a "surge" of okay feeling, and then I would think I was past whatever was going on. Wrong. The intervals between the cycling got longer, but the depression deepened rapidly. The rapid cycling deep depression is an animal of a different kind. It frightens me. I am terrified. The rapid cycling up-down is making me feel crazy. I can tell you that if people who are severely bipolar commit suicide, I now understand why—the rapid cycling really confuses my brain and sent me into a panic or deep depression. About 3:00 p.m. that day, I began to get panicky, so I took an Ativan, which eventually helped some. Around 7:30 I took another and went to bed. On Thursday I went back on Ritalin and was able to function at school but with difficulty. The cycling continued but not as often. I am better than I was when I first came but not nearly as well as I was on Monday. My head was hurting during the cycling—not a migraine—just an achy head. So I took the Hydrocodone, which did help me. Please make the cycling stop.
>
> Peggy

The English teacher can write! Her descriptions of the experience of rapid cycling bipolarity could not be done any better.

She told me that the discussion of sexual abuse was so anxiety-inducing that she would, in any other circumstance, have left the room, but her responsibility as moderator of the event would not let her. She was sure, she said, that the new medicine, Concerta, was the problem because her symptoms came on immediately after she had taken the first pill. She had discarded it and had returned to the Ritalin and on that drug felt at least somewhat better. I told Peggy I didn't think the Concerta, which is just a long-acting form of Ritalin, was doing it. I told her I thought it was the intense emotional trauma surrounding a lecture on sexual abuse that had precipitated her worsening. I encouraged a psychiatric consultation. She expressed ambivalence.

"I am getting better. My moods aren't shifting as much now, and I have discovered that with the Ritalin, I can take more Topamax without having as many flashbacks. That is helping my migraine. I am 80 percent of where I want to be. I am really not sure I need a psychiatrist."

"Okay, Peggy, but keep it in mind. I want you to increase your Ritalin, and I am prescribing a new drug called Abilify. It is a mood stabilizer. I am giving you some samples of 5 mg pills. That is a very low dosage, but with a little luck it will help."

On her next visit, Peggy told me "I am 100 percent there. I can only take one-half of the Abilify pill. More than that makes me sleepy. My moods aren't swinging, and I haven't had a flashback. Do you remember the rainstorm we had a few days ago? That would always make me have a headache, but this time no headache at all."

"That good, Peggy?"

"Yes, really that good. This is the first time I have felt well in thirteen years. No fibromyalgia, no headache, no flashback, no depression, no cycling moods."

"Well, Peggy, I hope it holds, but it sure looks like we have the right combination."

"There is one thing more. It is really strange, but I want to share it with you. I can now recall a time at age five when I was sexually molested by an older boy in the neighborhood. I guess I had repressed that all my life. Is it possible that these medicines have let me remember things that I had tried to forget?"

"Yes, Peggy, and this is not rare. I have seen it before. The right medicine restores the chemical balance in the brain, and memories that have been repressed can come to light. I must ask you, did that memory cause anxiety?"

"No, not at all. I feel complete now. I feel happy."

Peggy has maintained her wellness now for over a year. She told me on a recent visit that she had surgery on her knee, and this was the first time ever she had an operation without becoming depressed. We shared our experiences together as I scanned the chart. I called to her attention to the fact that we began her treatment on March 25, 2009, and essentially completed it on May 6 of the same year, the day I prescribed Abilify. In less than six weeks, an interval that included an episode of rapid cycling bipolarity, we had seen the end of bipolar depression occurring over forty years of her life. And with it cessation of mood shifts, fibromyalgia, migraines, and the flashbacks of post-traumatic stress disorder.

Russell was a talented guy, and his life was one of achievement. He was forty-nine years old and many years married with three kids. He was an artist specializing in miniatures and a personal trainer. In his spare time he sold and serviced aquariums. He was a licensed importer of tropical fish.

He was reluctant to talk about some of his past experiences, but clearly there was physical, if not sexual abuse from his parents, forcing him to be moved out of the home to live with his grandparents from age eleven on. The trauma notwithstanding, his life had been comfortable until, at age thirty-seven, he developed excruciating, crushing pain in his arms and legs. His doctors could find no cause, and is often the case with the undiagnosable strange illness, it was suggested he might have some form of multiple sclerosis. Among the drugs given him then was the anticonvulsant, Lyrica. He told me that this drug made him feel confused, and for the first time in his life he started flashing back to his father's beatings. That went away when he stopped the Lyrica. He took Hydrocodone for his pain, and after a year or so, it gradually went away. He did acknowledge that during his painful interval he was, for the first time, sleepless and depressed.

Russell remained well for some twelve years, and then his symptoms reappeared full force. That is when he came to me. Searching for some hint of bipolarity in his past history, I learned that he had always had high energy and had been subject to mind-racing and also intervals of great creativity. He denied mood shifts but acknowledged the recurrence of depression, insomnia, and flashbacks just like the first time he suffered pain. He told me, in response to my questions, that he did not suffer from bad dreams, but he did offer a good history of cataplectic attacks with sudden unaccountable falls to the floor because of weakness in his legs. He also offered an observation that I don't believe I had ever heard before. He told me that when he was most in pain, his memory and mental focus actually improved. I am used to people telling me they become angry, irritable, and mentally distracted with pain but never before had I heard of mental capacity improving with pain. I prescribed Klonopin and Methadone.

Another resurrection. Within twenty-four hours of starting the drugs, he experienced relief of pain and the depression. He was back to training and painting. He gave me two of his miniatures. The one painted before my treatment was dark-hued—purples, grays, and browns. The more recent was bright with scarlet, orange, and yellow colors.

Over the ensuing months, we did encounter a few issues. One was the gradual reappearance of pain and depression. This abated when I increased his Methadone dose. He continued, however, to have occasional cataplectic falls. This was most interesting to me. I had controlled virtually all the symptoms of his disease but could not get on top of the cataplexy. Still, I was pleased. A lot had been achieved. It was to last about a year, and then on a routine visit, he came in with his wife. He obviously was disturbed, and he let his wife do the talking. She told me he was having a lot more pain and depression, and the flashbacks had come back. She told me also that he was reluctant to tell me about this because I might think him a drugseeker. A few more questions, and I learned that his abusive father had a terminal illness, and Russell was the caregiver. I also learned that with his relapse, Russell was exhibiting a great deal of irritability and unprovoked anger. His drop attacks had increased in frequency. I increased the Methadone dose, and he recovered from pain, depression, and anger. His falling spells also diminished.

Another few months, and then another problem. A routine cardiogram used to monitor the Methadone effects on the heart showed a change. One of the intervals, that which measures the time between the onset of cardiac contraction and recovery from the contraction was increased. This was a hint that Russell was at risk for a cardiac arrhythmia, potentially fatal. More alarming was his complaint that he wasn't getting enough air, that he felt short of breath. That symptom in the opiate user always demands attention. I wasn't certain that my patient was headed for trouble, but there was at least a significant possibility.

"Russell, I know the Methadone has been a miracle drug for you, but I am afraid we are having problems with it. I want you to see if you can reduce the dose, and I am going to give you another opiate. It is called Oxycodone and will hopefully take the place of the Methadone. I don't know what is going to happen here, but this is something I feel we must do."

"Okay, it was my miracle drug, and I hate to lose it, but I will do what you say."

On his return, he told me he had tapered the Methadone and within several days totally discarded it. The Oxycodone, to his surprise (and mine), worked quite as well, if not better, than the Methadone. He told me the effect was not as sustained as with the Methadone, however, and that is what we would expect. Oxycodone is a quicker and shorter-acting drug than Methadone. I liberalized the dosage, allowing him to take it every four hours instead of the eight he had done with the Methadone. He later told me that he didn't realize how short of breath he really was until he got off the Methadone.

How close were we to a disaster, a cardiac arrest? I don't know, but I suspect it may have been a near thing.

Russell is now on Oxycodone 180 mg daily. A big dose, perhaps, in the minds of those not accustomed to prescribing the drug, but I have lots of patients who need even more. He has achieved near complete resolution of his symptoms. He no longer experiences pain or depression. His flashbacks have stopped entirely. Mental focus and energy are at a very high level, and most remarkably, his cataplectic drop attacks have finally stopped.

"Doc, I've got something to tell you. You know I am taking six of the Oxycodone pills a day. If I miss just one I start falling again."

"Does anything else bad happen when you omit one pill? Depression? Pain? Anything?"

"No, nothing except what do you call it—cataplexy?"

"Yes, cataplexy. You mean, if you miss only one pill, you start falling again?"

"That's correct."

Oxycodone prevents cataplexy. That makes no sense at all, that is unless you are accepting of the bipolar spectrum and opiate cure.

Let's compare Russell's illness with Peggy's. Both suffered childhood trauma. Russell seemed for a while unaffected by his, but Peggy evolved rapidly into post-traumatic stress disorder and bipolarity. It was only years later that both of them developed pain. Peggy's appeared, along with worsening of her bipolarity and PTSD, after a hysterectomy. I do not know why Russell's occurred. There was no obvious stressor. It just up and happened, but with it came, for the first time, flashbacks of his childhood abuse, this seemingly appearing under the sponsorship of the anticonvulsant, Lyrica. Peggy had a similar experience. The anticonvulsant, Topamax, made her flashbacks worse. I am not sure I have ever heard this kind of complaint before.

Russell and Peggy experienced, over the course of several months, diminution of pain and its attendants. Seemingly a spontaneous recovery. It does happen. Then years later, Peggy suffered recurrence of pain, worsening depression, mood shifts, and flashbacks after a bladder operation. Russell had a near-identical recurrence of his symptoms under the provocation of caring for his terminally ill, abusive father. Ultimately, both of them got well—Peggy with Ritalin and Abilify; Russell with Klonopin, Methadone, and later Oxycodone. With their recovery from pain and bipolarity, they also experienced arrest of their post-traumatic stress disorder flashbacks.

Both Peggy and Russell suffered through the course of their lives cyclic, recurring pain. Whether this cyclicity bears any relationship to the cyclicity of bipolar disorder, I do not know, but I do suspect there is a relationship.

Clay was nine years old when his grandfather, in a drunken frenzy, shot him and his younger brother. The brother died immediately. Clay survived and was able to witness his grandfather then taking his own life by slitting his throat with a straight razor. Homicidality and suicidality. Was Clay's grandfather bipolar?

He grew up to be a truck driver and go through four marriages. He told me it would have only been one if he had found his current wife first. He denied any problem with anxiety or depression but reported that he did frequently flashback and relive, tearfully, his childhood experience. At age thirty-five he began to experience back pain. An orthopedic surgeon told him that an operation would do no good. Within a year he began ongoing opiate therapy in the form of Morphine and Hydrocodone. At his age forty-five, two years before coming to me, he retired from his job and for the first time became depressed. He was given several different antidepressants and found Cymbalta the best. I told him to continue that drug, and I prescribed, in addition, Klonopin and Imipramine and maintained his opiate therapy.

Clay did about as well as I could expect under the circumstances. His depression and pain ameliorated, and he slept somewhat better. The flashbacks continued, however, but, strangely, they were less disturbing to him. There were the usual mishaps. He ran out of his Cymbalta, and within five days was profoundly depressed. On another occasion he ran out of his Morphine and suffered a withdrawal. Along the way I did routine urine drug tests, and they were appropriate for the drugs he was taking—Hydrocodone and Morphine and also marijuana, an agent that he told me was very pain relieving to him. I accepted what he told me, and never again in conversation with Clay did I reference the use of marijuana.

Interestingly, there is a component of marijuana known as Tetrahydrocannibinol (THC) that is FDA-approved as an antinausea and appetite-enhancing drug for use in people with cancer and HIV infections. Its trade name is Marinol, and probably unsurprisingly, it can occasionally be pain-relieving and mood-stabilizing.

Like several other patients presented in this book, I began seeing Clay before I learned about the bipolar spectrum, before I had learned what to ask and what to look for. Some two years into my care, he appeared looking particularly down and in pain. He told me his wife had a terrible outcome from Lasik surgery to correct her nearsightedness. She was in great pain and facing a corneal transplant. I extended my concerns and took the occasion to spend a little more time with Clay. He volunteered in response to my question that he was having a problem controlling his temper, and that he felt angry all the time. Also, he was having very strange dreams, some of his childhood event and some otherwise, just bizarre, strange dreams that were very threatening to him. He was sometimes paralyzed when he awoke from them. He was also experiencing daytime sleepiness.

Once again, the bipolar spectrum was emerging from latency under the provocation of stress. What had been chronic pain, depression, and post-traumatic stress disorder was becoming the bipolar spectrum. I added Ritalin and commented to him that we have the option, if that fails, of going to Methadone in addition to the other opiates.

"How are we doing now, Clay?"

He smiled and said, "It was like a lightswitch turned on. Everything was better in just a few days."

"Tell me everything about it."

"Well my pain is a lot better. That is the big thing I guess."

"What else?"

"I am not depressed anymore. I sleep much better."

"How about the dreams, the flashbacks?"

"They are gone! Totally gone. I am a different person. I am a happy person."

"That's great. I am thrilled."

"One more thing, Doc. Could you write me a prescription for Viagra?"

"More interested in sex now, Clay?"

"Yes, and I need a little help."

"Sure."

Recovery from pain can certainly be associated with restoration of sexual desire. It turned out that Clay, like others with chronic pain, even those doing well, get sick with other diseases. His was a blockage in the lower aorta causing impotence and leg pain when he walked any distance. He underwent surgical repair and did well.

I enjoy Clay's visits. On a recent one he asked me, "Dr. Cochran, do you ever watch The History Channel?"

"Yes, sometimes I do. It can be pretty good."

"Well, I watch it a lot, and they had a piece on Howard Hughes recently. I am sure you know about him. He was a pilot and businessman, and he made a fortune in the aviation industry."

"Yes, Clay, I know about that."

"Well you may know that he was in a plane crash and nearly died. He had chronic pain after that, and you will be interested to know that his doctors gave him Klonopin and Imipramine—the same medicines you started me on."

"That is very interesting. Let's just say he had some pretty good doctors."

Clay laughed, and then there were a few moments of hesitation as I began to recall a bit more about Howard Hughes. "You know Clay, if my memory serves me correctly, in his later years Howard Hughes became a recluse. He refused to touch other persons, to shake their hands. He was obsessed with the notion of germs, and I am rather sure he had obsessive-compulsive disorder."

"Hey, that's right Dr. Cochran. I remember that. They talked about it on the program. Does obsessive-compulsive disorder have anything to do with pain?"

"Yes."

Greta was twenty-nine and had chronic back pain due to *scoliosis* (curvature of the spine). She experienced her first sexual molestation at age nine at the hands of a neighbor and close family friend. There were other occasions and other girls. When they finally told, he was arrested and discovered to have video recordings of his sexual acts. He was sentenced to a long prison term.

At age twelve Greta attempted suicide by slashing her wrist. At age sixteen she began to have flashbacks. At age twenty-nine she required a psychiatric hospitalization for suicidality and was diagnosed with bipolarity. Following that, she came under the care of a new psychiatrist, one expert in the treatment of bipolar disorder. When she came to me she was taking

Zoloft, Xanax, and the sleep aid, Restoril. Her moods were reasonably stable on this program, but she continued to experience terrifying flashbacks. Her most common trigger was a smell but also sometimes an image of one reminded her of the attacker. She also suffered vivid dreams, some of her remembered experience but others, as she described them, were "off the wall." She would be quite fearful on awakening from these and also intensely painful in her back. With a few, she had experienced sleep paralysis. She acknowledged mind busyness and distractibility. She told me she had "too many thoughts," and that her psychiatrist suggested that she might have attention deficit disorder. On top of it all, she had migraine that didn't respond to triptan therapy. Her headaches would last a day or two, and she was experiencing about two per week.

"That's a remarkable history, Greta. You have been through a lot. How are your moods doing now?"

"I am depressed. I am tired of feeling bad. I feel sad and hopeless."

"Any thoughts of suicide now?"

"Not now."

"What are you taking for pain?"

"Nothing right now. My orthopedist gave me some Hydrocodone, but that made me sick at my stomach. Then he gave me some Oxycodone. That helped, but he didn't want to keep giving it to me. I think that's why he referred me to you."

"Did your orthopedist suggest that you were a candidate for surgery?"

"Yes, but I am unemployed and have no medical insurance. I don't think I could stand an operation anyway."

A good candidate for Methadone, I thought, and I prescribed it up to 10 mg every eight hours. She tolerated it poorly with nausea and itching and was not able to take it for sufficient time to note any benefit at all. I had the option of going to a psychostimulant because she did have features of narcolepsy and ADD. I elected instead to resume the Oxycodone in a higher dose than her orthopedist had been willing to provide. I told her she could take 15 mg four times daily.

She told that she was getting substantial relief, and that her mood was better. She was not as mood-shifty and was also becoming more social, going out with friends, and she was quite pleased with that. There had been no change in her headaches, however. I told her I was very encouraged, and we would simply push the dose up to 90 mg daily. I wrote in my notes that I was witnessing the mood-stabilizing and antidepressant effect of an opiate, and I made sure to copy that to her psychiatrist.

"I am doing a lot better on the bigger dose of Oxycodone. The back pain is much better, and I am not nearly as depressed. My headaches are also improving."

"How about the flashbacks, and how about the problem with distractibility?"

"Both are a lot better. Really, I am a lot more cheerful than when I first saw you ten months ago."

"That's wonderful, Greta. You are doing so well I don't think I need to see you for another three months. By the way, are you still seeing your psychiatrist?"

"Yes, and he is very happy with the way I am doing, I don't have to see him for another six months."

"That's wonderful news. Let me ask you, what does he say about the Oxycodone? Does he relate your improvement to Oxycodone?

"I am just not sure. He doesn't seem to want to talk about it."

"Well, you are better, and I am very pleased. I will see you in three months."

On Greta's next appointment, she volunteered that the flashbacks were beginning to come back. She was feeling more anxious and depressed. It began, she told me, when she learned the man who had abused her was, after eighteen years in prison, being released. I told her that I thought this would be a short-term thing, and I would like to wait it out for now, but if it was necessary, I could increase her Oxycodone therapy. She told me that her counselor had said the same thing.

A brief review. I have presented you the case histories of four people who suffered childhood abuse and post-traumatic stress disorder. They all experienced the near total cessation of flashbacks on my therapy. In two, it was with psychostimulants, and in two with opiates. I made those treatment choices according to what I thought, under the circumstances, to be the drug most likely to benefit. It would be interesting to know if those who responded to stimulants would also respond to opiates and vice versa. Attempting that experiment would, however, be unconscionable. My patients were doing quite well, and I am happy to leave things the way they are.

Another point, both Peggy and Greta were diagnosed and treated by psychiatrists for their bipolar disorder. Clay and Russell were never diagnosed with bipolarity by a psychiatrist, and almost certainly would not have been had they seen one. Nonetheless, I am sure that they were soft bipolars, and their dramatic response, one to Ritalin and the other to Methadone and later Oxycodone, confirms, at least to my mind, that diagnosis.

A few months before this writing, a patient gave me a newspaper clipping concerning the high incidence of post-traumatic stress disorder in military personnel injured in the Near East. The military had conducted a study and found that the combat wounded who received Morphine within an hour or so of the injury had a much lower incidence of later post-traumatic stress disorder than those who did not receive Morphine early on. Morphine for stress disorder. Interesting.

Before concluding this chapter, I want to tell you briefly about a patient who touched me deeply.

Randy was a young man of purpose. He was a college graduate and a firefighter, having risen at a very young age to a captaincy. I listened to the story of his achievements because many with chronic pain tell me the same tale—how a life of satisfaction and reward had been so totally undermined by chronic pain. His began with a motor vehicle accident in which his back was injured. On imaging studies, his doctors could find no certain cause for his pain. He was advised that watchful waiting was in order. He was prescribed the opiate, Oxycodone. With this drug and the passage of time, he improved a bit and was able to go back to work until one day, while on duty, he experienced sciatica, intense pain in the back radiating into the left leg. He was taken to his physician's office where he was given an injection of the opiate, Nubain. Within but moments, he experienced a great increase in both his back and leg pain and with it sweats, chills, tremors, abdominal pain, nausea, vomiting, and diarrhea and also confusion. He remained in and out of delirium for several hours until he awoke in the emergency room slowly becoming lucid and able to comprehend.

Nubain is one of a few opiates that have an *agonist/antagonist* effect on opiate receptors within the brain. In plain speak, this means the drug will stimulate some opiate receptors but will simultaneously block others. That is what happened in Randy's brain. The effect of the Oxycodone he had been taking was immediately inhibited because its receptor was blocked by Nubain, and he entered a sudden opiate withdrawal. To put this in some perspective for you, very few people die of opiate withdrawal but many wish they would. And that refers to, shall we say, a natural opiate withdrawal. If a person is withdrawn from a long-acting opiate, withdrawal will come later and will probably be milder. With a shorter-acting drug, the withdrawal appears more rapidly, but never as rapidly as Randy experienced. His was an artificially induced withdrawal, and it was immediate and total. It staggers the mind to think just how bad that experience could be.

"I would rather die than go through that again. It was horrible. The worst thing that has ever happened to me."

"That was several months ago, wasn't it Randy? What has happened since then?"

"They say I have post-traumatic stress disorder. I keep flashing back to it. I relive it sometimes when I am awake and sometimes in my dreams also."

"Are there triggers?"

"Yes, many triggers. I will flashback when I see things that remind me of an emergency room. Seeing a gurney or hypodermic syringe or even a picture of them will cause me to flashback."

I pursued my inquiries. I was particularly interested in the nature of his original accident and whether he might have been rendered, however briefly, concussed and unconscious. Concussions can be a harbinger of chronic pain.

"Randy, let's go back to that accident again. I know your back was injured. Did you have any other injuries? Did you strike your head? Did you lose consciousness?"

No answer. I looked up from my note taking at Randy. He was mute. His jaw had dropped. His face was devoid of any animation or expression. His gaze was into the distance, and tears were welling up in his eyes, and all this occurred in a matter of seconds. His wife, in attendance, had obviously witnessed this before. She went over to him, took his hand, and stroked his neck lightly and said, "I love you, honey. This will go away soon."

And it did. In a short while Randy was restored and able to resume conversation. I asked, I'm afraid with great insensitivity, "What was that?"

"A flashback."

"I'm sorry, Randy, if I said or did something that provoked this, and obviously I did, I apologize."

"That's okay, it was when you used that word, *consciousness*. That triggered it."

For the first time in my over fifty years as a physician, I had witnessed, actually seen with my own eyes, what a flashback does to a person. It must be, and many of my readers are probably aware of this, a horrible experience.

I never saw Randy again. I thought we had a good interview. I thought sooner or later I could figure out some way to make him better. He didn't come back, and I don't know why—or maybe I do. It may have been an insurance issue. Maybe he came to surgery and got well. Maybe he found a smarter doctor. I really don't know, but I have the suspicion that maybe, just maybe, I became a trigger. Could he be avoiding me because he fears another flashback? Speculation to be sure but not without precedent. Think about panic disorder. If a woman suffers a panic attack while shopping in a shoe store, she will be very reluctant to go into that store again for fear she might suffer from another panic attack. This avoidant behavior is self-protective, a very natural thing to do.

Randy, if you read this book, let me tell you that you taught me a lot, and I hope you have recovered.

CHAPTER 8

Attention Deficiency

Sue was troubled with chronic neck pain. She had consulted several orthopedists but none found any evidence of major problems. She was forty years old, unmarried, tattooed, and at the time of her first visit, an unemployed laboratory technician. I noted from her intake history that she was on Klonopin and Adderall. I use that combination not infrequently, but very few people come to me on it.

She told me that she grew up in a very dysfunctional home and began to experience depression in her teens. She had been under psychiatric care and over the years had taken a great number of different antidepressants, mostly SSRIs. She told me that most of them would work for a while and then suddenly lose their effect, which required change to another drug. Among the other medicines that she had been given were Depakote, Tegretol, Zyprexa, and Abilify—all mood stabilizers.

"Let me ask you a question Sue, those kinds of drugs are often used for the treatment of bipolar disorder. Did your psychiatrist discuss that with you?"

"No, he kind of skirted that issue. He did say one time, I remember, that I had a tendency to bipolarity."

"Do you have mood shifts? Are you up and down?"

"Yes, some, but always with my menstrual period. I get very bitchy."

"Do you ever get speeded up, hyperactive, or do you have intervals where you get very agitated?"

"Yes, that does happen some."

"Are you still depressed?"

"Yes, I am depressed almost all the time."

"Sue, this may seem a strange question, but I need to ask it. Do you have problems handling your money? Do you go on spending sprees or buy things that you don't need?"

"Yes, that really has been a problem for me. I don't allow myself to carry a credit card."

"How is your sleep?"

"It is very poor."

"Do you dream?"

"Yes, but most of them are good. Only occasionally do I have a bad one, and those can upset me very much."

"I see that you are taking Adderall now. Could you tell me what that is for?"

"My psychiatrist diagnosed attention deficit disorder about eight years ago, and I have been on the drug ever since. It really does help my mental focus and attention."

"Tell me about it."

"I was a poor student, and I had to work extra hard to do my schoolwork. I couldn't seem to keep my mind on any one idea. Let me tell you something interesting, Dr. Cochran. Before I started the Adderall, when I really tried to concentrate, when I had to maintain mental focus, I would suddenly get very sleepy, so much so that I would have to pinch myself to wake up."

"Thank you for sharing that with me. That is most interesting."

And it was. I marveled again at the interconnection, the links between ADD, narcolepsy, and bipolar disease. These disorders and the symptoms they engender simply don't fit in a box. They form a continuum, a spectrum.

"Did the Adderall help your depression?"

"Not really. But my psychiatrist has just started me on Cymbalta, and I like that a lot. I think it is the best drug I have ever taken, but it keeps me from having an orgasm."

"Let's leave that problem in the hands of the psychiatrist, Sue. Let me ask you about the Klonopin. How long have you been on that?"

"I started that just a few weeks ago. I had been on Ambien, but I started sleepwalking on that, so Dr. Smith gave me Klonopin. It works much better."

"Have you ever been given an opiate for your pain?"

"No, none of my doctors have ever offered me any painkilling drugs other than Darvocet, and that doesn't do anything."

"I am going to write a prescription for Methadone. It is a pretty good painkiller, and I think it may help in ways that you don't expect. I certainly don't know for sure, but it is worth a try."

"Oh, I am kind of scared of Methadone. Could we try something else?"

"We can if you wish, but there are good reasons for trying the Methadone first."

"Okay, as you say. What do you think it is going to do for me? Will it help my pain?"

"I hope so."

She returned three weeks later, and when I walked in the room she was smiling. I could tell immediately that she was better, but I could not keep my eyes from dropping. She was wearing a low-cut blouse, and the full extent of her tattoos was quite evident. They consisted of arabesque figures extending from between her breasts toward each shoulder. Interesting, I thought, but time to get to business.

"How are you feeling, Sue?"

She laughed and said, "Wonderful."

"What is wonderful?"

"Everything."

"Tell me about it."

"Well, my pain is almost gone and my depression also. I stopped the Cymbalta about a week ago."

"What else?"

"Well my sleep is good, and my mood is even. I didn't get bitchy and irritable with my last period. I just feel happier now, happier than in a long time."

"How much Methadone are you taking?"

"Just like you said, a pill three times a day."

On the next visit she told me she had a new job at an industrial laboratory, and she was very excited about that. I wrote a prescription for Methadone and told her to return in a couple of months.

"Dr. Cochran, could you write me a prescription for Fiorinal?"

"Well, you have to tell me why you are taking Fiorinal."

"It is for my migraine. I've had a real problem with headaches, and I have taken Imitrex and all those other drugs like it, and none of them work for me. One of my doctors gave me a prescription for Fiorinal several years ago, and it is an absolutely perfect drug. As soon as I feel a headache coming on, I take one, and the headache just vanishes."

"How often do you have a headache?"

"Oh, maybe two or three times a week, but it is not a bother at all as long as I have my Fiorinal. I couldn't get by without it."

"I'll be happy to write it for you."

Fiorinal is a combination of the barbiturate, Butalbital, caffeine, and aspirin. It has been around for over fifty years, and Sue's response to it is a reminder that older (and cheaper) drugs can be quite as effective as the newer ones. Most of the recoveries that I tell you about in this book came with very old drugs. Just a reminder.

When Sue returned, she presented an arresting image. My eyes dropped once again to her rather daring yellow blouse and her tattoos. She was wearing large loop earrings, crimson satin boxer shorts, black fishnet hose, and high heels. Ostentatious habit to be sure, particularly so in one who, after leaving my office, was going to work at a chemical laboratory testing asphalt. I have mentioned before and will again that adornment is often the bipolar way.

She came early for her next visit with an interesting story to tell. She loved her new job but found it very demanding, and she was beginning to experience problems with focus and attention. It wasn't sedation, she told me, just that her mind "wanted to shut down." She said it was different from sleepiness.

Thinking that Methadone was the culprit, she discontinued the drug and within days, the pain, depression, and insomnia all reappeared. She then did something that human beings, particularly bipolar ones in pain, are wont to do. She experimented with her medicines. She gradually doubled her Adderall dose up to 120 mg and resumed the Methadone. On that combination she was restored.

What Sue did was dangerous and irresponsible and also, regrettably, the bipolar way. I scolded her, telling her that drug adjustments must be done with my knowledge. In my heart, though, I knew it was a futile exercise because those in pain know the dosage of the drugs they need to control their symptoms. I gave her new prescriptions in the requested amount, and I cautioned against a too-rapid escalation, but I remained servant to the observation that my patient was better, and that, in the end, is always the determinant.

Hazel was a thirty-eight-year-old nurse's assistant who had a lumbar fusion a year before. Pain, however, persisted. She entered the care of a pain clinic and was given Hydrocodone. She had a falling out with her pain doctor and then was referred by her orthopedist to me. She offered a long history of depression and related that she has been on many antidepressants. Two of them, Celexa and Zoloft, made her worse. She denied suicidal ideation except for one interval four years before when she and her husband separated. I found nothing in the initial interview to suggest bipolar disease. She did tell me that the Hydrocodone gave her a measure of comfort and also was energizing to her. I accepted this observation because it does happen frequently. I prescribed it for her at the requested dose, 10 mg four times daily, and also Klonopin to help her sleeplessness. I instructed her to continue her current antidepressant, Cymbalta, which she told me had been helpful. I scheduled a return appointment, as I usually do, in three weeks.

My nurse took a call but ten days later. Hazel told her that she had to use more of the Hydrocodone than prescribed and asked what she could do about it. My nurse advised her to come in immediately. She complied, and I got an entirely different picture the second time around. She told me that she had had bad experiences with pain doctors before, and that she was quite fearful of me. She was afraid, she said, to tell me the whole truth. She had been taking eight Hydrocodone a day instead of the prescribed four, and this was the reason she was discharged from her prior pain clinic. For several months she had been overusing the medicine because there was simply no way she could work and raise her children without the pain-relieving and energizing effects of the Hydrocodone. She also reported that when she ran out of her pain medicine, she became not only painful but sleepless and subject to mind-racing and anger.

"Hazel, why did you lie to me?"

"I'm sorry, Dr. Cochran, but I have a problem with trust. I have never had a doctor that I felt I could trust. I've always felt like I was being accused of being an addict, a drug-seeker. Will you forgive me? Will you help me?"

"Yes, but I demand your candor with me. Believe me, I know what you have been experiencing. Most of my patients have been accused by their doctors of drug-seeking. I understand your dilemma, but we do have a problem. You must limit your Hydrocodone to six pills daily. As you probably know, every formulation of Hydrocodone contains Tylenol, and you are taking too much of it. I am going to to help you though. I am giving you a new drug called Methadone. Take it with the Hydrocodone and come back to see me in three weeks."

Her response to Methadone was quite interesting. She took a single pill, felt very sedated on it but slept well that night, and the next morning was considerably better with much diminished pain. She took another pill and started feeling short of breath. This recurred every time she took a pill, so she discontinued it.

Again, shortness of breath with opiates. It was quite appropriate that she stop the drug, but, in its own way, it had helped her for a while at least by restoring her sleep. Her response, sedation and breathlessness notwithstanding, was another clue to bipolarity. She was ever more forthcoming. She continued to report that the Hydrocodone helped her pain and also her mood. She felt more even on the drug. She found it very calming, and under intervals of stress she would often reach for her pain pills. She emphasized that with the Hydrocodone, she could wake up in the morning, take her shower, go to work in the emergency room, and perform very effectively. In the absence of her pain medicine, she couldn't do this because of daytime somnolence and depression.

I told her she might be a candidate for psychostimulant therapy, and then she told me that several years before she was diagnosed with attention deficit disorder and was given the drug, Adderall. She said it was very disagreeable to her. It made her feel unwell, like her hair was standing on end. She then volunteered that in the past she had taken the appetite suppressant Phentermine, and she found that drug very helpful. Not only did she lose weight, she felt emotionally much better. She thought it helped her attention deficiency. Nonetheless, it was ultimately discontinued because of her doctor's concern of heart damage with the long-term use of that particular drug.

"Hazel, why didn't you tell me about the diagnosis of ADD? You know that was important for me to know. Why didn't you tell me?"

"I'm sorry. I told you I have a problem with trust. I am fearful of telling people, particularly doctors, about myself. I know they will take it the wrong way."

"Get over it, Hazel. We've got work to do. I'm going to give you another opiate, Oxycodone, in addition to the Hydrocodone. We will continue the Cymbalta and the Klonopin.

She reported clear improvement, not only in pain, but also mood and energy. Her major problem was nocturnal pain with awakenings throughout the night, and this occurred even if she took her opiates at bedtime. We talked some more about the Phentermine, and she reported that it was mood-stabilizing, and that it diminished her thought-racing and inattention. She told me that even her mother-in-law, who hates her, said she was more even on the drug.

Phentermine is derived from amphetamine. It was developed and marketed as an appetite suppressant. Its role in the treatment of attention deficit disorder and other psychiatric diseases has, to my knowledge, never been really explored. Nonetheless, it *could* work in the same manner that Ritalin and Adderall do, and she was not the first person who has told me about the mood-stabilizing and attention-restoring effects of Phentermine. One of the difficulties of Phentermine is that with long-term usage, there can be damage to the heart valves, and for that reason it is usually prescribed over the short-term, maybe for a matter of a few months. I elected to employ it as a *therapeutic trial*. In this case it was just to see what would happen, to see if it was as good as she said it was. With that knowledge obtained, I could pursue other options. I prescribed it in low dosage.

She reported great benefit with arrest of inattention, mind-racing, and stabilization of mood even beyond what she had achieved with opiate therapy. Moreover, her nocturnal attacks of leg pain had disappeared. She became more open with me and related that several years ago, when she and her husband were separated, she did "some disinhibited behaviors." I asked what they were, and she said "sex and drugs." I told her to continue the Hydrocodone, Oxycodone, Klonopin, Cymbalta, and Phentermine. We were still within the interval of time when that drug was reasonably safe. Satisfied with her progress, I gave her a prescription for a month's supply of her several medicines. She told me she was going to see her new primary care doctor soon.

I saw her at the appointed time, and she told me that her new doctor had demanded that she stop the Phentermine, telling her that it was dangerous for her heart. Contrary to his instructions, however, she had continued it and now had exhausted her prescription. What to do? I prescribed Ritalin starting at 10 mg daily and going up to 30 if it did not disagree with her.

She reported that the Ritalin was even better than the Phentermine, and in fact for the first time in years she felt "normal." She was taking more than I prescribed, however, and I encouraged her not to freelance with her drugs in the future. I reminded her that she had a history of doing this. Nonetheless, the patient knows the right dosage. They know how they feel. I prescribed up to 50 mg daily.

We got several months out of the Ritalin and the other drugs, and then she began to develop headaches and disposition change. She reported that she felt "mean" when she took the Ritalin. I instructed a progressive taper. The results were predictable. She developed distractibility, thought-racing, depression, and reappearance of severe pain awakening her at night. When that happened, she would immediately take a Hydrocodone and lie in agony for forty-five minutes before its effect took hold.

I wrote a prescription for Vyvanse. It is like Adderall but in the form of a *prodrug*. That is to say that its actual molecular configuration has no pharmacologic effect, but within the body it is metabolized, that is, changed into Amphetamine, which is Adderall. Why it should work better than Adderall I am not sure, but it did and without any of the hair-on-end effects.

She told me that the Vyvanse stopped the "strobe light in my mind." She was having absolutely no cravings for more Hydrocodone. She was energized and very happy in her work in the emergency room. The conversation then turned to an issue that I think was very much with her.

"Dr. Cochran, I don't know if I am an addict or not. I know I was fearful of the opiates, but I had to have them to function. Do you think that makes me an addict?"

"No, I think you are a person who had not been given the right dose of the right drugs."

"You know, we see so much drug-seeking in the emergency room. People come in requesting drugs and tell all kind of lies to get them. They even bring their children with them and rehearse the kids to say the right thing. I am not sure our doctors treat those people very well."

"Are you sure, really sure, that they are drug-seeking, that their complaints are not legitimate?"

"Well, I am pretty sure, but you are right, I am not completely sure."

"You lied to me to get drugs, didn't you?"

"You are hurting me, Dr. Cochran."

"Good. You are hurting those people when you presume they are drug-seekers."

"I see what you mean."

"Have you ever gone to an emergency room to get drugs, Hazel?"

"No, I have never done that, but I will admit some of my friends have shared their medicines with me. I feel very guilty about that, but I am also very confused. I must tell you I am more tolerant of the patients we see in the emergency room now, but I really don't know how many of them are seeking drugs for pleasure or really seeking relief of pain."

"Hazel, sometimes I think we would have less drug abuse if we used more, not less, of the drugs. I think we tend to ration them to our patients. That is what happened to you. You took more than prescribed, but I don't think that necessarily makes you a drug addict. I think that makes you a person who was undertreated."

Several years back while skiing in Colorado, I injured my knee. It was swollen and quite painful. Friends carried me to a local emergency room, and I introduced myself as a doctor to the physician on duty. I told him of my prior history of knee trouble. He was very kind. He took an X-ray and satisfied himself that there was no fracture. It was a ligament injury that could await my return to my regular orthopedist. I thanked him and told him that I really was having a lot of pain, and that I had used the opiate, Meperidine, with some previous knee injuries and asked if he would be willing to provide that. His demeanor changed suddenly and totally. My request had angered him, and he became hostile, telling me he would under no circumstances give me anything stronger than a Tylenol and Codeine combination. It didn't help at all.

Jennifer was a forty-one-year-old nurse with back pain for which she was taking Hydrocodone. Her medical history was, sadly, typical. She was severely traumatized as a teenager—kidnapped, raped, and beaten. She required facial and dental surgery and entered long-term psychiatric care for post-traumatic stress disorder. She also, in the past, suffered "terrible migraines." She had been intolerant of triptan therapy and reported that when she was given injections of the opiates, Nubain or Stadol, for her migraine, she experienced severe rage. She had a strong family history of bipolarity and attention deficit disorder, and she described mood shifts and spells of mind-racing and talkativeness. She also acknowledged, in response to my question, that she had gone on spending sprees several times that resulted in considerable financial stress for her family. She volunteered that she often wondered if she had attention deficit disorder. She made pretty good grades in school but had to work very hard to get them. She suffered postpartum depression after each of her three children was born.

I maintained her Hydrocodone therapy and added Methadone. She was the perfect candidate for the drug for she suffered chronic pain and, probably, bipolarity. I was particularly interested in her reactions to injections of Stadol and Nubain. They produced rage. That, I believe, is a clue to bipolarity. Moreover, she had a positive family history and also the specter of childhood trauma and post-traumatic stress disorder, neither of which I can dissociate from bipolarity.

Her response was sudden and total. Pain was diminished and mood stabilized. The only downside was a couple of intervals of sleepwalking, an experience she had not known before. She didn't seem particularly disturbed by it nor was I. We would just put up with a little sleepwalking for a while. I increased the dosage of Methadone knowing that she would find the right level.

Later, a phone call from her. She was developing swelling in her legs and hands, a not uncommon problem with Methadone. I told her to discontinue it and to return to me as soon as possible.

Her swelling had diminished, but mood shifts and pain, unresponsive to Hydrocodone, had returned full force. I gave her Oxycodone and told her to resume the Methadone in low dosage but to discontinue it if the swelling reappeared.

On her return, she told me the Oxycodone did not help her pain, but with the resumption of Methadone three times daily "my mood has really evened out." Mood stabilized on Methadone but with no pain control. I prescribed Morphine.

She didn't tolerate the Morphine, and she continued to have pain in the back. Her mood, she kept emphasizing, was stable on the Methadone and Hydrocodone and, fortunately, her sleepwalking had terminated. I chose another opiate, Hydromorphone (better known by the brand name Dilaudid). She didn't tolerate it because of sedation. She had failed Oxycodone, Morphine, and Hydromorphone for her pain. She and I together explored her options, and she told me that although the Oxycodone had been ineffective for pain, it had produced no side effects. I gave her a larger dose than before, and she prospered. She told me that Oxycodone and Methadone were the best combination ever. She was having less pain and was using the Hydrocodone only for occasional breakthrough pain. She had even gone back to work as a home health nurse. She told me she was enjoying it enormously.

She came in early for her next visit saying her son had stolen her medicines. I was upset to say the least, and I demanded some kind of explanation. She told me her son was brain-injured and had major behavior problems. He had been in jail many times for altercations and thefts.

"Is your son bipolar? You do have a strong family history of the disorder."

"He has never been diagnosed with bipolar disorder, but I am sure he has it."

"Okay, Jennifer, I am going to work with you because we have found a real good combination of medicines for you. You have been restored, you are back at work, and I don't want you to lose that, but you will lose it unless you manage these medicines better."

Was Jennifer telling me the truth? Somehow, I believe she was. But she was going to continue to test me.

"Dr. Cochran, I am still doing good, but I have got a problem. I don't know exactly what is causing it, but I have become very careless. I am having problems with my record-keeping at work. I am easily distracted, and I can't finish tasks anymore."

Faced with a new problem, I responded as I always do by reviewing the entire medical record to see what might have been missed along the way.

"Jennifer, when you first came in, you told me that you wondered if you had ADD. You told me you made good grades in school, but you had to work hard to get them. Tell me more about your symptoms. What were they like back then, and what are they like now?"

"Well, they are pretty much the same. Dr. Cochran, there was something I didn't tell you. I was diagnosed with ADD when I was a teenager, and I was given Adderall for it. I couldn't have gotten through college without that drug, but then I just gradually got better. People do outgrow ADD don't they?"

"Yes, they can, but why in the name of heaven did you not tell me that you were diagnosed and treated for attention deficit disorder? You had plenty of opportunity to do that because we talked about that issue. I am having trouble, Jennifer, with your lack of candor."

"I don't know why. I really don't know why. Maybe I was ashamed of it. Maybe I thought it was unnecessary. Maybe I thought that it would just make it more difficult for you."

"Jennifer, I ought to fire you. You are a nurse, you know these things are important. Nonetheless, I am willing to give you some Adderall."

"Thank you, Doctor. I think it will help me. It did before. You have stuck with me, and I appreciate it, but I have one more problem that I hate to tell you about."

"Go ahead and tell me, I am ready for it."

"A month ago you gave me two prescriptions for the opiates. I got the first filled and then lost the other one when I washed it in the pocket of my jeans. That is why I am in early."

The pain doctor has to put up with a lot of lies. We have seen that a lot, haven't we? I have learned, and I have tried to example this throughout this book that many of these lies are an attempt to accommodate to fear, distrust, and the rightful need to find the appropriate dose of the appropriate medicine. I am more tolerant of this behavior than I used to be, but Jen was pushing me absolutely to the limit, and I had to employ a process that

I usually eschew. I had to stand in judgment of her. I don't like that. I like treating my patient, not judging them.

"Jennifer, I am not going to give you the Adderall yet. I have to be sure of your compliance, and you haven't been very good at that. I will give one-month prescriptions for your Methadone, Oxycodone, and Hydrocodone. I want you to return then, and we will again think about the Adderall."

I hated that I was being so judgmental, so punitive, but there was no recourse.

One month later she presented me with the "washed" prescription. She had forgotten that she had actually saved it so that she could present it to me. Forgotten? Well, maybe her attention deficit disorder did need treating.

"Jen, I am glad you found the script and brought it to me. That helps restore my trust in you. Now let's get down to work. Are you still having trouble with mental focus?"

"Yes, it is getting worse. I am not sure I can continue working."

"Your mood, your sleep?"

"Perfect."

"Adderall it is. Start on a low dosage and build up to 20 mg if you tolerate it. Here is another month of the Methadone and Oxycodone."

What was going on here? Was her distractibility and inattention due to her opiate therapy? Probably not. Her symptoms were much more typical of ADD than of a drug reaction, although the latter cannot be totally counted out. Moreover, she had a past history of treatment for the disorder. Why it should eclipse for twenty years or so and then reappear when she was getting well from the rest of her bipolar spectrum I do not exactly know, but as I have written before, the symptoms of bipolarity can appear and reappear at different times in our lives.

"I am normal. I see it, and my family sees it. They can all tell the improvement. I suspect I have had attention deficit disorder for a long time. Maybe I had so many other problems that I didn't think about that."

"How much Adderall are you taking?"

"Just like you said—20 mg."

"Do you feel that you need more?"

"Well I would like to try more just to see."

"You can go up to 30 mg."

"Could you give me some extra Hydrocodone? The weather is getting cold now, and I always have more pain in the cold weather. I have been using the Hydrocodone just occasionally for breakthrough pain, and I would like to have a little more on hand."

I complied. Her complaint is a common one—pain worsening in colder weather. Besides, the increase in her opiate therapy was trivial considering her dosages of Methadone and Oxycodone.

It has gone well with Jen for nearly a year. Our visits have lost their urgency, and I have enjoyed the opportunity to reflect with her on the events of her life. She tells me that she is remembering more of her childhood, and that she was having fewer flashbacks of it. She also tells me that on the anniversary of the month of her abduction she usually became very depressed. Not so this time. She also told me she was attending Al-Anon meetings to help her cope better with her bipolar son's drug and alcohol abuse.

Jennifer and Hazel were both nurses. They thought they knew the way the medical world operates. They believed they had to lie to me to obtain the necessary care. They did not trust me, but I trusted them. With time my trust was rewarded by their recovery.

It is trust, perhaps above all else, that those in pain need and deserve, but I am afraid they don't always receive it, either from their doctors or their nurses.

Linda was fifty years old, thirty years married with two kids. Her pain began twelve years before. Originating in the low back, it spread throughout her body, and she was diagnosed with fibromyalgia. She was using Darvocet for pain. I learned that simultaneously with the onset of her pain, "my emotions took over." She became extremely anxious and depressed and began seeing psychiatrists. She was told that he had bipolar disorder. Along the way she was given several drugs including Zoloft, Paxil, Risperdal, Zyprexa, Seroquel, and Lithium. At the time she came to me she was taking Wellbutrin and Lyrica, which did diminish her discomfort somewhat. She was sleepless and described occasional vivid dreams but no problem with daytime sleepiness. She did tell me that there was a close parallel between her pain and mental focus. The more she hurt, the less well she could think and remember. She had a son with attention deficit disorder and also a nephew.

"Dr. Cochran, I am sure your patients have told you about fibro fog. You do know what I am talking about, don't you? I have a lot of friends with fibromyalgia, and they all say the same thing—that they just can't think and remember."

"Yes, I hear that a lot. I am going to introduce an idea to you, and that is that fibro fog is actually adult attention deficit disorder. Does that make any sense to you?"

She hesitated for a few moments and then said, "You know I never thought about it that way, but that is what my son has, and I guess that is what I have."

"You have been told that you have bipolar disorder, and that was several years ago. What were your emotions like back then?"

"Mostly down and depressed but sometimes with periods of irritability and anger."

"You have been given several bipolar drugs. Among others, you have taken Lithium and Seroquel and also some antidepressants. How did you react to those?"

"Not very well to the antidepressants, and for that matter, the other drugs, the mood stabilizers, didn't help me much. Lithium was pretty good for a while but eventually its effect wore off, and I am taking Wellbutrin now."

"Are you still mood shifting?"

"Yes, some, and still a lot of irritability, but I am better than I was ten years ago."

"Are you still seeing your psychiatrist?"

"Yes. Dr. Rogers has really helped me."

"Linda, let's go back to when you first became painful. Was anything going on in your life? Were there stressors—financial, martial, or whatever?"

"No, none that I can really remember. It just seemed to have kind of come over me."

"From what you have told me, it seems that your depression and your pain came on pretty much the same time. Is that correct?"

She paused and then said, "You know, they really did. Just within a few months of each other. I never made that connection before. Do you think there is a relationship between the two?"

"Yes, almost certainly. Linda, let me ask you this. Have you talked to your psychiatrist about your fibro fog, your inattention and distractibility?"

"Yes, I did, but she didn't seem very concerned about it. Do you think it is important?"

"Very. I am going to start you on stimulant therapy. The name of the drug is Adderall. I want you to start at a low dose, just a half a pill a day and build up to two pills daily."

Why was her psychiatrist dismissive of her complaints of inattention and distractibility? I don't know for certain, but I suspect she believed that her patient's impairments were modest, and that treatment would entail the addition of yet another drug, a stimulant, one with the capacity for side effects and addiction and perhaps even the induction of mania. Again, the measure of potential harm against probable benefit. To return to a theme noted earlier in this book, it is the breadth of the bipolar spectrum and its many different expressions (symptoms) that allow us so many points of attack. Treat *every* symptom because in doing so you can sometimes cure the patient.

She was smiling when she came back. "Dr. Cochran, I am doing a lot better. I am taking the Adderall twice daily, and my thinking is better. I am not as scattered in my thoughts, and I have actually started reading a book. I haven't done that in a long time. Something else, after talking with you I realized that the Darvocet I was taking for pain was actually helping my mood. Is that possible?"

"Yes, quite possible. How are you doing with the pain since you have been on Adderall?"

"A little bit better. The Adderall seems to make the Darvocet work better, but I am still having a lot of pain, and I am not sleeping well at all."

"Linda, I am going to increase your Adderall dosage. You are taking 20 mg now. You can work your way up to 40 mg. I also want to give you a stronger pain pill. It is Hydrocodone, and the preparation has some Tylenol in it, just like the Darvocet. I want you to try it, and if it is better than Darvocet, go ahead and use it. If not, go back to the Darvocet, but I don't want you to be taking the two drugs together at the same time. That will be too much Tylenol."

She liked the Hydrocodone but found that the Adderall was making her a little more nervous, so she had to reduce the dose. Nonetheless, she reported that her mood had progressively stabilized, and that she had become "less critical." Her husband and family also saw it. This comment was most interesting to me. I have already written that the successfully treated bipolar employs such descriptors as "even," "level," and "balanced." Other descriptions I often hear relate to the improvement in disposition. Linda told me she was not as critical. Other expressions I hear are "I am more patient," "I am more tolerant," "I'm not as angry," and even "I'm more empathetic." Like level, even, and balanced, these kinds of expression come almost exclusively from the successfully treated bipolar.

Sandy was thirty-eight years old, married, and working with her husband in an insurance agency. She suffered abdominal pain. It came on after gastric bypass surgery. The benefit from the operation was remarkable. Weight loss was achieved easily but at the price of recurring pain. It would come and go and was worse when she was physically more active. The more she did, the more she would hurt. It would often flare at night, and she would try to relieve it by placing an icepack on her abdomen. Sleep was impaired, and she acknowledged mind racing at night. She described vivid dreams, most of which were quite pleasant. Occasionally, however, they were very frightening to her and were associated with a sense of paralysis when she awoke from them. She had been diagnosed as bipolar when she was a teenager and had seen several different psychiatrists. Currently she was taking Topamax, which was helpful in reducing her mood swings and also her recurrent migraine. Nonetheless, she reported intervals of depression mixed with "grumpy spells." I asked her if she had experienced mania in the past, and she said that she did, and that it was "phenomenal, but it usually makes me do things I shouldn't do." She acknowledged daytime sleepiness and having to struggle to stay awake. She complained of severe fatigue since the onset of her pain and also forgetfulness and distractibility. She told me that one of her therapists suggested she might have attention deficit disorder. I prescribed Adderall and told her to continue taking the Hydrocodone that she had been given for pain.

"Dr. Cochran, I am euphoric. When you saw me three weeks ago, I couldn't even walk to the mailbox. Last weekend my husband and I were reinstalling doors, putting in a new mailbox, and getting a lot of other things done around the house."

"Keep talking. Tell me everything."

"I have a lot more energy, and my mental focus is much better. My mood is more even, and I have almost no pain at all. I am happy. I really feel good."

"Okay, Sandy, this is good news, but I hope my medicine hasn't made you manic. You seem to have a little bit of that in you. You know what mania is like. Is this mania?"

"No, this isn't mania."

"Okay, you can experiment, Sandy. I am going to write a prescription for up to 30 mg of the Adderall from the 20 mg you are taking now, try to find you a level, and be on the watch for mania because it can happen."

I have written before about emotional euphoria in the bipolar. Sandy had told me that her mania was a phenomenal experience. Realize that recovery from pain and bipolar mood shifts can also be a pretty phenomenal experience. Maybe Sandy was a little bit manic, but a little manic is not a bad place to be. It invites achievement and creativity. If my patients end up just a little bit manic, or better hypomanic, that doesn't bother me at all.

"Dr. Cochran, I am much more active now, and I am afraid I am having more pain. Except for the pain, I am doing well. My mood is even, and my mental focus is great. But the pain is back, and I am having to use more Hydrocodone. Can you okay an early refill for my pharmacist?"

"Yes, I'll have my nurse call and tell him you can get the prescription filled early. I am going to add a new opiate—it is called Methadone. I want you to take one pill, 10 mg three times daily. If you feel that you need to take less, that is okay with me, but I don't want you to take more. Back in three weeks."

When she returned, she reported some distressing news. Just a week after she last saw me, her brother and her favorite niece were killed in an automobile accident. Her brother immediately, her niece later, on a ventilator, declared brain-dead.

"But her heart is still beating. She was an organ donor. Eleven people! Can you believe that, Dr. Cochran. Eleven people received tissue from her."

"That is amazing, Sandy. I suppose that gives you some closure if that is possible."

"It is sort of a closure. Dr. Cochran, I could never have survived this without your medicines."

Back to the task at hand. "How are you doing with the Methadone?"

"It nauseates me a little. I can only take a half a pill at a time, but I am thrilled with the pain relief."

"Let's stay where we are, Sandy. I will give you a month's prescription for the Adderall and Methadone. I want you to know I am available if you need to come back sooner. You have been through quite a trial, and you seemed to have handled it well. I don't want things to get ahead of us, though."

I reflected on Sandy and all that had happened to her. She had been under my care for three months, and I had witnessed her resurrection with Adderall and later Methadone and the survival of the emotional trauma of losing loved ones. It was too good to be true, and as is often the case, it was. She returned but three weeks later, complaining of a new pain, this in her chest. She had relapsed into more depression, anxiety, and sleeplessness. I suggested an increase in the dose of Methadone, and she told me half of a pill three times a day was all she could take because of nausea. I gave her Oxycodone in a pretty big start-up dose, 15 mg four times daily.

"The Oxycodone has really helped. It has taken the Topamax to a new level."

"What do you mean by that, Sandy?"

"You may not believe this, but I have more common sense now than I used to. I can think better. I am not depressed, and my pain has gone away, absolutely gone away."

Well, I suppose "I have more common sense" stands up there with "I'm less critical," I'm more patient," and "I am more empathetic." It is still hard for me to believe just how well these people who suffer from bipolarity and pain can actually do, just how much can be achieved.

We must, however, keep our feet on the ground. Much was indeed achieved in the people I describe in this chapter but at the price of the simultaneous use of a stimulant and an opiate, sometimes several opiates. And there is really nothing wrong with that at all. At least until some circumstance forces them to an emergency room or a new doctor where they will almost certainly be labeled as drug-seeking addicts.

CHAPTER 9

Obsessions

Carly visited my Web site and thought I might be able to help her. The ostensible problem was numbness in her hand and pain that awoke her throughout the night. The carpal tunnel syndrome can usually be relieved with surgery, but Carly was a self-employed real estate broker and had no medical insurance. She could not afford the operation. Her physician gave her Hydrocodone, which, astonishingly, relieved everything.

Her obsessive-compulsive disorder had been present, she told me, since her teen years, but it was only diagnosed at her age thirty-two. She also suffered depression and was given, over the course of many years, a variety of drugs. When she came to me she was taking Paxil and Wellbutrin and also Amitriptyline prescribed some months before for her migraine.

She told me she obsessed about something terrible happening if she deviated from ritual. Walking on patterned surfaces such as tile floors or brick walkways was very distressing to her because she knew if she did not step on the appropriate tile, her mother would surely die. Thus, a misstep provoked extreme anxiety. She was also a counter and a toucher. When she entered a room, she felt obliged to count every object and touch those within reach. If she was unable to do so, she became quite anxious. And never, she told me, did she leave her home without hand sanitizer in her purse.

Remarkably, over the course of fifteen years, her depression and her OCD would alternately wax and wane. When depression was her predominant symptom, her obsessions and compulsions diminished, and when her obsessions were predominant, her depression lessened. I can only speculate as to why this happened. I suppose that when the depression was bad and the brain was tired, it didn't have the energy to obsess, and when obsessions were bad, the brain was so full of intrusive thoughts and fears that it didn't have time to be depressed. Regardless, hers was a fascinating story of alternating obsessive-compulsive disorder and depression throughout her life. It was in this setting that she developed carpal tunnel syndrome and, with it, extravagant pain.

This brings us to the Hydrocodone. Within hours of taking it, she told me, she felt an unknown calmness and well-being. Fearful, anxiety-producing obsessions abated and her depression also.

"I couldn't believe it was happening. It was too good to be true. I couldn't wait to tell my psychiatrist."

"I think I know where this is going to go. Keep talking."

"He was totally dismissive of the idea that Hydrocodone could do what it did to me. This angered me, and I will admit, I got a little bit testy. I told him I wasn't a liar, that I wasn't making it up, and that I was simply sharing something important with my doctor. After all, he had been working with me for years, and I wasn't doing very well at all. Why not try something new?"

"Well, it doesn't surprise me that the psychiatrist would be hesitant to use opiates for the treatment of your disease, but that doesn't give him the right to disparage your observation."

"It was worse than disparagement. He told me that if Hydrocodone made me feel that good, I was on my way to becoming a drug addict. I left his office crying and angry, very angry. I went on the Internet looking for information on Hydrocodone and mental illness, and that was when I found your Web site. Are you willing to give me the Hydrocodone?"

"Yes, I will prescribe it 10 mg up to six pills daily. You will probably know when you are at the right dosage. You might as well remain on the Wellbutrin and Paxil. I will take over prescribing them."

She reacted to Hydrocodone just as she had before—arrest of obsessions and depression. She required the full dosage for the effect, and she told me that the Hydrocodone was energizing her and keeping her from sleeping. I added Klonopin, and she prospered.

"Dr. Cochran, there is something happening that is really interesting to me. Because my mind has been so full of thoughts, I have always had trouble reading and comprehending. I can't retain the material. Now with the Hydrocodone I am able to read your book, which is the first book I have read since college."

I continued to see Carly for about a year, and she had life's usual ups and downs. A breast cancer scare but also an exciting job in the music publishing business. She also suffered an extremely painful kidney stone attack. Her urologist told her she could just take extra Hydrocodone. She did, up to twenty pills daily! There is probably nothing really wrong with 200 mg of Hydrocodone a day, but in the process she was taking ten grams of Tylenol, far above the recommended maximum of three grams. Fortunately, the liver function tests that I performed were within normal limits. She had been undamaged by her experience, but she well could have been.

Many of my patients are taking opiates in combination with Tylenol. They often express their concerns over liver injury. I try to reassure them because I don't think I have ever seen a real problem when the medications are taken as prescribed. Ten grams, however, is way too much, and Carly escaped what could have been a disaster.

Carly moved away to another state, but when I last saw her, she was having no pain and had required no surgery for the carpal tunnel because it was asymptomatic. She was no longer depressed, she no longer suffered unwarranted fears, and she no longer had to touch things.

Jack was a newspaper reporter. Some two years before he came to me, he developed back pain and, with it, increasing difficulty with painful urination. His voidings were frequent, some six times each night. The diagnosis of *interstitial cystitis* was made. It is but another form of chronic pain, and like so many of them, the cause is uncertain. The urologist prescribed Amitriptyline and Oxycodone up to four times a day, and then referred him to me.

I learned that he was sleepless, and his worst bladder pain would occur about four or five in the morning. He had to void very frequently. If he held his urine, the subsequent voiding would be bitterly painful. He acknowledged some anxiety and depression for the past two years, and he volunteered that he had become kind of obsessive-compulsive. He found himself worrying excessively about things he had no need to worry about. He also reported that with his sieges of pain, he would get down and feel very depressed. He told me both his father and sister suffered depression, but that there was no bipolar disease in the family.

I was excited about treating Jack because almost never do I see a male with interstitial cystitis. It is much a female-predominant disease. I maintained his Oxycodone and gave him Klonopin to take at night along with the Amitriptyline.

"Dr. Cochran, I am taking the new medicines just as you prescribed, and they are doing nothing. My urination hurts just as bad—it may even be worse, and I am still waking up all through the night. Can we try something else?"

"Continue the medicines as before, and I am going to give you a different opiate called Methadone. I want you to take it with the Oxycodone."

On his next visit he again reported no change. He had discarded the Klonopin and Amitriptyline, and he was obviously getting more and more frustrated.

"Jack, I am almost certainly going to find a way to get better. Don't give up hope. I am going to rewrite the Methadone. You have been taking one pill every eight hours. I want you to gradually increase the dose, and you can go up to three pills every eight hours. I am also going to give you Xanax because you seem rather anxious to me."

"Oh, am I!"

The next time I saw Jack he looked better. He was taking the Methadone as I prescribed, 30 mg every eight hours, and said his pain dropped from 7 or 8 on a 10 scale to a 4 or 5. I wasn't sure how much of his improvement was due to Xanax and how much was due to Methadone, but I was very happy with our progress.

As time went by, Jack became more open with me. He told me that throughout his life he has been subject to mind-racing and obsessive worry—not about anything in particular, just whatever attracted his attention at any particular moment. He also told me that he was diagnosed with attention deficit hyperactivity disorder as a child, but his mother did not want him to take Ritalin.

Jack is now eighteen months into treatment. His nocturnal voidings have reduced in number to three. They are not nearly as painful. We reflected on the course of his illness in recovery, and I told him that only recently have I become more tuned to the frequency of obsessive-compulsive disorder in those in pain. I confessed that my interrogations regarding that issue had not been as detailed or thoughtful as they should have been. Then I asked if there was anything else he wanted to tell me about his OCD and ADD.

"Oh, by the time I got to you I thought I was going crazy. I was embarrassed about it, and I didn't tell you about it, but I was always in a cleaning frenzy. It is really strange, I was afraid to look down to the floor or the ground. I feared that something bad was going to attack me like a snake or spider or something. I also had to carry a water bottle with me all the time. I couldn't be without my water bottle. I could not stand to not have it."

"Thought-scatter?"

"Yes, terrible thought-scatter. Like I told you, I thought I was going crazy."

"And that is all gone now?"

"All gone."

The confluence of OCD and ADD and their cure, along with the pain, by Methadone.

Devona was a fifty-four-year-old career woman. She had a long history of migraine and had been on treatment with Topamax for many years. In 2006 she was in an automobile accident and suffered a neck injury and a concussion. It left her with inattention, distractibility, and problems with speech. She stuttered and frequently had problems finding the right word. She received intensive speech therapy for several months following the accident. She improved but continued to have problems with word finding, especially late in the afternoon when she was tired. She also continued to have neck pain and with it the appearance of *allodynia*, that is, the perception of pain in response to trivial sensory stimulation. Wearing a necklace was painful to her.

Following her accident, her headaches changed. Formerly episodic migraine, they became an incessant dull generalized pain. This is the disorder formerly and even now described, lamentably, as *tension headache*. As I have written many times before, the patient does not have a headache because she is tense. She is tense because she has a headache that no one knows how to treat. The condition can be more appropriately described as transformed migraine, and I have referenced that before. Her episodic migraine pain was, under the influence of head trauma, transformed into an unremitting headache.

After a couple of years of intermittent physical therapy and epidural steroid injections in the neck, she came to a surgical fusion. It did not significantly help her pain. She was taking Hydrocodone in a fairly low dose. She offered a long history of psychiatric care for the treatment of anxiety and depression. She had been taking Prozac and Xanax for most of that time. More recently she had been given the stimulant, Strattera, from her psychiatrist. She found it helpful for her mental focus and word finding.

Most physicians would recognize Devona's illness as the *postconcussion syndrome*. Others would recognize it by the name of *traumatic brain injury* (TBI). Few would suggest it was attention deficit disorder. We do not usually think of that as being derivative of trauma, but it is interesting that her psychiatrist chose the drug Strattera. It is indicated for the treatment of ADD, and it helped her. Interesting also that difficulty with word finding is, at least in my opinion, a very frequent complaint among those who suffer from ADD.

"Devona, your medical history is most interesting. I guess our big problem, the reason you are here to see me, is your neck pain and headache. Is that correct?"

"Yes, but there are some other problems too. Since my accident, I have been having very scary dreams. Also, I find my moods shifting, and several of my friends have told me that sometimes I talk too much."

"Did the mood-shifting get any better when you were started on Strattera?"

"A little, but it is still a problem. And there is another problem I have had for a long time. I think I have obsessive-compulsive disorder."

"Have you talked to your psychiatrist about it?"

"Yes, but he doesn't seem to think it is much of a problem. And maybe it is not. It is just a part of me that I don't particularly like."

"Tell me about it."

"Well, I am a hand-washer, and I do a lot of repetitive acts like closing doors and turning doorknobs. I have to do it four times. If I don't, I feel very anxious."

"Do you do mental repetitions like counting things?"

"Yes. I talk to myself, and I say the same thing over and over."

"What do you say?"

"May the Lord bless and keep you, may his countenance shine upon you and grant you peace. May the Lord bless and keep you, may his countenance shine upon you and grant you peace. May the Lord bless and keep you, may his countenance shine upon you and grant you peace. May the Lord bless and keep you, may his countenance shine upon you and grant you peace."

"That was four times, wasn't it? Is that when you usually stop?"

"Usually I go much longer, but I always have to stop on an even number. I feel unsettled if I don't."

"Did the Strattera help control any of your OCD symptoms?"

"Not really."

"I am glad you brought this OCD thing up. I do see a pattern here. You have attention deficit disorder, obsessive-compulsive disorder, and maybe a hint of narcolepsy. Vivid dreams are very common in that disorder. Do you get sleepy during the day?"

"Yes, I do, and it is becoming more of a problem."

An interesting evolution. A depressed, obsessive *migraineur* (one who has migraines) who was concussed in an automobile accident and then developed attention deficit disorder and impaired speech. On top of all that, a hint of bipolarity with mood shifts and talkativeness and narcolepsy with vivid dreams and sleepiness. There is a continuum.

Would all this give me a clue about how to treat her pain? What could I do that the psychiatrist hadn't done? I knew where I was going to go with this, but I started off with conservative and conventional therapy. I prescribed Imipramine and Klonopin, and I liberalized her Hydrocodone.

"I like your medicine. I am certainly sleeping better. I am not having the dreams, and my pain is better since you gave me more Hydrocodone."

"And the depression?"

"I think that is better. My mental focus also. It is still a problem, but it is better. There is no doubt about it."

"And how about the OCD?"

"It hasn't changed a bit."

I was pleased with her progress and a little bit surprised that so many different things improved with very conservative therapy. I elected to stay the course and see her again in another month.

"How are you doing Devona?"

"I am better. I want you to know that you have helped me, and I appreciate your efforts, but I am not where I want to be. The pain is still there, and I am still mood-shifting and talking to myself. You have helped my sleep, and I can't tell you how grateful I am for that."

"Devona, I am willing to get a little more aggressive here, and I am going to intrude on your psychiatrist's care. I will inform him of this by sending him a copy of my notes. I work with the man a lot, and I think he will be willing to accept my suggestions. I want to give you the stimulant, Adderall. If it gives you any difficulty, particularly if you feel nervous or tremulous or you feel your heart racing, I want you to stop the drug immediately and call me. I am looking forward to seeing you again in two weeks."

Strattera is a pretty good drug for attention deficit disorder, and it lacks the addictive potential of the psychostimulants. That attribute makes it rather attractive to prescribers. Devona's psychiatrist had given her the safest drug but, in my opinion, not necessarily the best. That is the reason that her improvement on it was incomplete. Again, a case of measuring the potential harm of the drug against the probability of benefit.

She could hardly contain herself when I next saw her. "It is amazing. It is absolutely amazing. I cannot believe it!"

"That good?"

"Yes, unbelievable. I have more energy. My mental focus is better. I don't stutter at the end of the day, and my pain is a lot better. My headaches have almost gone away. I am so grateful."

"Any down side to the medicine? Is it bothering you in any way?"

"No, not at all."

"Have you talked to your psychiatrist?"

"Yes. He said he was happy with what you are doing. He said I could just stop the Strattera."

"Is anything happening to your OCD?"

"Yes, a lot. I don't talk to myself as much. My door-closing compulsion has slowed down quite a lot."

"Devona, I am thrilled. We will stay where we are, and I will write you a two-month prescription for Adderall. Continue your other medications."

It was four, not two, months later when she returned. She told me that she reduced her Adderall dose by half. She was taking only 5 mg twice daily, a miniscule dose, and was getting by just fine. She told me she had received a promotion at work and, quite happily, was also losing weight. I told her that was probably an Adderall effect although that certainly was not my intention in prescribing it. But no harm done so long as the weight loss does not become extreme.

A year into her care with me, Devona continues to do well. She did have a setback, though. She was displaced from her home and her medicines when the floods hit Nashville in May 2010. It was time of discombobulation. She was unable to reach me for more prescriptions. She was out of her medicines, all of them, for some two weeks. It all came back—the pain, the depression, the mood shifts, the dreams, and the repetitive benedictions.

Sometimes when medicines that are working are suddenly stopped for whatever reason, their resumption does not always give the benefit that they formerly did. It is a fact of life. Thankfully, however, it didn't happen. When Devona got back on her medicines, everything settled down.

Kate has only been under my care for a couple of months. Too brief a time, probably, to render a judgment on the ultimate outcome, but she is a textbook case in the study of chronic pain, the bipolar spectrum, and the opiate cure. She was thirty-eight, twice married and divorced. She had two children, aged sixteen and twenty. She suffered low back pain for many years and came to her first operation, a lumbar fusion, a couple of years before coming to me. It actually worsened her pain, which began radiating down the left leg. A second operation was necessary, and although her leg pain was relieved, her back continued to hurt, worse than ever. Her surgeon prescribed Oxycodone and referred her to me.

The interview was difficult. Her speech was rapid and her thought scattered. She was very restless, constantly changing her position and sometimes standing up to pace back and forth across the examining room, all the while tearfully lamenting her fate.

She was raised in a military family and sexually and physically abused by her father. This was repetitive and, she acknowledged, accounted for her getting married at age seventeen to get away. At her age twenty-seven, she became very depressed and anxious and entered ten years of off-and-on psychiatric care. Among the drugs she took were Xanax, Lexapro, and Cymbalta. None had really helped her, and she had given up on psychiatrists. She suffered post-traumatic stress disorder and frequently flashed back to her childhood experiences. She also had vivid dreams, always of her father, and she was sleepless in part because of her pain and in part, she told me, because of her inability to stop the thoughts racing through her mind. She told me she was easily distracted and had great difficulty carrying a task to completion. She also described mood shifts, suddenly becoming quite angry.

I completed the interview knowing that I had left a lot of meat on the bone. As time went by, I would surely find more. But for now, Imipramine and Klonopin and an increased dose of the Oxycodone. I commented in my consultation note that my restless and agitated patient was *catastrophizing*, that is, she was incessantly vocalizing her despair and hopelessness.

She returned but two days later. She was obviously distressed, hyperactive, and restless. Her thoughts remained scattered.

"Dr. Cochran, you just have to do something. Your medicine is not helping me."

"I am sorry, Kate, but we have only been at it a couple of days. I think I can get you better, but it is not going to be done in two or three days."

"I am so worried that I am never going to have a life again. I can't turn off my mind. The thoughts keep racing. Can I have some Xanax? Will that help my nerves? The Klonopin is doing nothing."

"I will give you Xanax, Kate."

"I want to try some Pristiq. I have read good things about that on the Internet. Can we start that?"

"No, Kate. I know you don't want to hear this, but we can't do everything at once. You are going to have to work with me on my agenda. You need to understand that."

"I'll try. I promise you I will really try," she said as she started wiping off the countertop with a moist paper towel.

She decided to come back just four days later. She was still crying and lamenting her fate—that one so young should be so sick. I told her that I was going to increase the Oxycodone and add a second opiate, Methadone. At least I was doing something, and that seemed to placate her. She volunteered to me that she was alphabet soup. She has been diagnosed with PTSD, OCD, ADD, and GAD (generalized anxiety disorder). I told her we could probably put a little BP (bipolarity) in there too. She didn't seem offended. With prescriptions for two opiates in her pocket, she left telling me that my medicines had made her no worse.

In only seven days, I had seen her three times, and I felt I had learned a lot. We were at least on our way.

"The increased Oxycodone does help. It really helps the pain, but the Methadone made me itch and didn't seem to help any. I have stopped it."

"Are you getting anything besides pain relief from the medicines—the Oxycodone and the Xanax?"

"They do seem to slow my mind down."

"That's good, that is what we want. I am going to increase the dosage, and I will see you again in three weeks. By the way, Kate, you don't seem as frustrated and anxious as you have been. You seem to not be as worried. Is that correct?"

"Yes. For a long time it seemed I really couldn't think about anything except the pain. It is not so bad now."

On our next visit, Kate and I really got into some interesting conversation. She told me that the Oxycodone and Xanax together was the best drug combination she had ever had. She also told me that her OCD was better. I asked her to give me the details of her symptoms, and she told me that obsessive cleaning was a part of it. She was also a counter, obsessively and repetitively counting the canned goods in her pantry and the books on her bookshelves. She arranged them so she could end on an odd number. An even one was "too perfect and just not right." She was obsessed with organization and neatness and told me that the vegetables were placed in her refrigerator according to their color—green next to yellow, next to orange, next to red. She told me that her obsessions and compulsions had diminished greatly on the Oxycodone and Xanax.

We talked some more about her childhood experiences. Her sexual and physical abuse was repetitive beginning at age ten. Her flashbacks, she told me, were always to her father's rapes. I asked her what her triggers were. She told me a movie or some reminder of an abusive situation would make her flash back, and also an image of a man who looked like her father would trigger. Interestingly, the sight of a military base would sometimes do the same. She volunteered that the flashbacks had became much less frequent and intense since being on the Oxycodone and Xanax.

Alphabet soup. PTSD, OCD, ADD, GAD, and BP. They all got better with a couple of drugs. There is a continuum.

Renee was referred to me by her orthopedist. She had some low back pain, but he did not think she needed an operation. I obtained a history of several years of depression. Along the way she had taken Wellbutrin, which made her more depressed, and Cymbalta, which made her feel "weird." She had been on Amitriptyline for several years for migraine, and that drug was pretty effective in preventing the headaches. She was taking Hydrocodone in low dosage for her pain, and it was becoming progressively unhelpful.

"Renee, does the pain stay the same all the time or does it come and go?"

"Oh, it definitely comes and goes. I will have waves of it sometimes lasting a week at a time."

"Do your moods change when you have the pain?"

"Well I am not sure that it is exactly with the pain, but I do periodically get feelings of being real energized. I feel kind of panicky when that happens, and I feel like I want to get out of the house and run."

"Anything else happen?"

"Yes, sometimes when I am that way, I get real irritable, and I just can't turn my mind off. I just keep getting flooded with different thoughts. Sometimes I can take a Benadryl or an extra Amitriptyline, and that helps. I really don't know what it is, but I don't like it."

"Do you have an anger problem, Renee?"

"Yes, sometimes I feel real mean. It just comes over me."

"Anything else?"

"Yes, I simply can't control my feelings. My emotions are a rollercoaster. Can you help?"

I was sure Renee suffered the bipolar spectrum. I prescribed Klonopin and jumped right in with Methadone.

"It is really working! My moods are much better. They are not shifting anymore. I am very pleased."

"How about the pain?"

"It is still there. It may be a little bit better, but I do have one problem, and it has been with me a long time. I don't think we talked about it much before, but I have these waves of fatigue. I just feel weak. I have no energy."

"Do you get sleepy when that happens?"

"No, just fatigued."

What a clue! Fatigue is a part of chronic pain and very probably other segments of the bipolar spectrum. It is not an uncommon complaint at all, and it offers us another point of attack. The pharmacy for chronic fatigue is a mixed bag. Some of the more stimulating antidepressants such as Wellbutrin can be used and also Provigil and Strattera. I much favor the psychostimulants, however, and I prescribed Adderall for Renee.

"I like this combination Dr. Cochran. I like it a lot. My fatigue is better. I have much more energy, and I am not on an emotional rollercoaster anymore."

"How is the pain doing?"

"Well, really not very well. The Methadone seemed to help at first. In fact, when I first took it I could tell in just a few hours that my pain was better. I have lost that effect now. Dr. Cochran, I hate to ask you this, and I don't want you to think ill of me. I want you to trust me, and I don't want you to think I am drug-seeker, but I really need some pain relief."

"I do not believe you are a drug-seeker. I recognize that you, and a great many of my other pain patients, have been made to feel that way. Chronic pain is a guilt trip, and opiate therapy makes it an even worse guilt trip. I hate that you people are so subject to prejudgment. I am willing to give you more pain medicine. Don't be afraid to ask me for it. You will know when you are on the right dose. Let's go up on the Methadone to 20 mg every eight hours. Continue the Adderall as before unless you feel that you need more. If you do, I will prescribe it."

"Thanks, Dr. Cochran. Thank you from the bottom of my heart. I think the Adderall is fine, but I do need more pain medicine."

Surprisingly, the increased Methadone didn't relieve her pain. She continued to report good control of her unstable moods, saying she no longer felt mean and no longer said things that she shouldn't. I increased the Methadone again.

"It is just not working, Dr. Cochran. I'm sorry, but it is not. I know you said you would give me more medicine if I needed it. I don't know what to do."

She had achieved, suddenly and totally, recovery from her mood swings, irritability, and anger with Methadone and Adderall but almost no relief of pain. What to do? Increasing the Methadone dosage was not a very attractive option to me. I do recognize that there is a threshold, a dose at which all symptoms are relieved, but occasionally Methadone (and other opiates) makes pain worse. I thought that might be happening. I elected to go to another opiate, adding Oxycodone, and telling her that she could experiment and actually try to take less Methadone. Perhaps the two opiates simultaneously could help her.

"It is perfect. Absolutely perfect. I did what you told me. I took the Oxycodone and reduced the Methadone. I am on the Adderall just like before, and everything is better."

"Well, Renee, what has happened to you is a bit unusual, but I have seen it before. Methadone controls your mood and your emotions but was unhelpful for your pain. I am glad the Oxycodone is working for that and, let me remind you, you are not taking too much medicine. You are not a drug-seeker."

"Thank you, Dr. Cochran. That means a lot to me. By the way, if you have time, I would like to tell you something that I think you will find interesting."

"Sure."

"We have never talked about this, but I have had a problem that really is embarrassing to me. I am a hair-puller. I guess it is just a habit that I can't break. I try to pull it from different parts of my scalp so it won't show so badly, but sometimes it does. It is very embarrassing to have a hairstylist call my attention to it. I used to respond to them with some excuse or another, but then I got to where I just didn't say anything. What I wanted to tell you was that as soon as I got on that Methadone, my hair-pulling stopped. It just absolutely suddenly stopped. I feel no need at all to do it since we started the Methadone. Thank you. You helped me in many ways."

"Thank you, Renee, you have helped me too. I have learned a lot from you."

Trichotillomania is the scientific name for compulsive hair-pulling. It is not uncommon, at least according to my patients who are hairstylists. I want to suggest that it may be an expression of obsessive-compulsive disorder. That is very much at variance with the diagnostic tables, and I am referring to the *Diagnostic and Statistical Manual of Mental Disorders,* published by American Psychiatric Association. That text states explicitly that trichotillomania is a disorder distinct from obsessive-compulsive disorder. Well, perhaps, but at least the authors recognize that there is enough similarity between the two conditions to address the issue.

If Renee's trichotillomania was not an expression of OCD, why did it go away with Methadone?

When I complete a book, the stories of those in pain must end. Their lives do not end, however. I want to reintroduce a person I wrote about in *Curing Chronic Pain,* and explore the remarkable evolution of her illness to address once again the phenomenon of catastrophizing.

Her name was Lucy, and her story begins on page 98 of *Curing Chronic Pain* in the chapter "Remembered Pain." I encourage you to reread it if you have a copy. If not, I will offer a synopsis and then tell you what has happened in the three years since her story was published.

She was an obese fifty-year-old who had a total of five back operations through her thirties and forties. Each gave her benefit until another disc ruptured. She was referred to me because she was again in pain, and this time her surgeon could find no ruptured disc, no cause for her pain. She told me through tears that she saw no hope for the future. Heretofore the surgeon had always found something he could fix. Now he couldn't, and she was sure she was destined to live a useless and painful life. She was repetitively vocalizing her despair. She was catastrophizing.

I prescribed Imipramine and Klonopin and later Lithium, empirically, because her sister and mother were bipolar. She improved very slowly with diminution of pain and despair, but her recovery was so slow that I suspected it was unrelated to my medications. Over the course of several years, she evolved into a very curious pattern of experiencing the same symptoms and behaviors she did when I first saw her. This occurred annually, almost always in the month of October. She would become very depressed, sleepless, and bitterly painful, and in a very stereotyped manner, resume the same incessant lamentations. On one of these occasions I added Topamax, the mood-stabilizing anticonvulsant, and she prospered—this time quickly. For the first time I thought I was seeing a true pharmacologic effect from a drug I administered her.

She felt well enough to proceed with gastric bypass surgery, which was quite successful. With weight loss, she had become a very attractive woman, and I was not surprised to learn that she had remarried after ten years of living alone. But then a problem with the Topamax. It is one of the few neuropsychiatric drugs that is an appetite suppressant, and it was maliciously so in her. She continued to lose weight at an alarming rate, and the Topamax had to be stopped. She did well without it—at least for a while.

It was at this juncture that I completed *Curing Chronic Pain*, and I am sharing with you the conclusion of Lucy's story from it.

> "Lucy's pain was, I believe, the recrudescence of the remembered experience of recurring back injury kindled over two decades. But why did it occur only periodically? What brain force was exciting into expression every October? I don't know, but I will offer a speculation. Lucy had a strong family history of bipolar disease. Moreover, her pain was cycling in the manner that depression and mania cycle in the bipolar. Is it possible that she did have bipolar disease, clinically silent for most of her life, but finally expressing itself as periodic attacks of remembered pain, sleeplessness, and a behavior pattern characterized by obsessive worry, anxiety, and the expression of hopelessness? Maybe it wasn't really bipolar disease, but it was certainly something like it."

A few months after these words were published, Lucy had another flare of her back pain. At the instigation of her sister, an operating room nurse in a major hospital in another city, she traveled there to seek a second opinion. She was told that a lumbar fusion would be curative. She underwent the operation and had more than her share of postoperative problems with respiratory depression and a wound infection. It took several weeks of antibiotic therapy to get it under control, but ultimately it was. When she returned home she came to see me and reported that the operation had benefited her. She was using an occasional Hydrocodone and getting by quite nicely.

The next October, it all reappeared—the back pain, sleeplessness, depression, and incessant worry with agitated expressions of doom and hopelessness. She was catastrophizing once again.

"I want to try the Topamax again. That was the drug that made me better. Can I try it again?"

"That's fine with me, but we will have to be vigilant to weight loss. I am writing you a prescription, and I am going to give you some more Hydrocodone for your pain. With luck, this thing will pass pretty quickly. Come back in three weeks."

She was still crying and lamenting when she left.

When I saw her next, I knew immediately that she was worse, not better. She was still catastrophizing, but there was something more. It was speech press. She was talking rapidly and forcefully, and her thought was scattered. She couldn't keep her mind on one subject for any time, and she knew it.

"I can't think. I can't remember. I can't control my thoughts. I know I am talking fast, but sometimes I just lose speech. I can't find the right word to say."

The bipolar spectrum in the form of mania and ADD was emerging right before my eyes. I elected to give her Ritalin, not an altogether bad choice but maybe not a good one. Maybe I should have tried a mood stabilizer, but she was already on Topamax. I told her to return in two weeks.

"The Ritalin has cleared my mind. I can think clearly now."

She was speaking rapidly but without tears this time. She told me that her memory had become acute. She was remembering more of her childhood, even the birth dates of kids she knew in grade school.

"Dr. Cochran, there is something I must tell you. I should have done it before, but I just wasn't sure about it. I am now. I remember it clearly. I was sexually abused several times when I was nine years old. It was by my uncle. He came to visit our family every October after he harvested his tobacco. He slept in an upstairs bedroom next to mine, and he would come in at night, get under the covers, and put his hand between my legs. I remember it, and I remember the smell, the smell of tobacco."

She was still speaking rapidly, and she had more to tell me.

"Dr. Cochran, I have brought all my medical records from my operation, and I want you to read them. I want you to read them right now. I need your help."

"Lucy, that stack of paper is an inch high, and I do not have time to read that now."

"Well, here, you keep them and read them as soon as you can. It is very important to me. I am afraid my sister is going to lose her job because of the problems I had after my surgery."

"Lucy, you are telling me that your sister is going to be fired because you got a postoperative infection. Is that right?"

"Yes, I am sure of it, and I need your help because I want to do everything I can to protect her."

Oh boy! This woman is in the middle of a manic episode and getting paranoid.

Next Lucy's husband. "Dr. Cochran, the family thinks that the Ritalin is making her talk too much. Lucy called her daughter past midnight and spent three hours on the phone. She can't seem to stop talking. All the family sees it. We think it is due to the Ritalin. What do you think?"

"I know I am talking a lot, but I have a lot on my mind. I have a lot of things I have to talk about."

What a pickle I was in! I had a patient who was in bipolar mania, perhaps made worse by my therapy with Ritalin. But it had cured her attention deficiency and restored her memory. What to do?

The first order of business was to get an appointment with a psychiatrist as soon as possible. Until that time, she was to reduce the Ritalin from 20 mg to 5 mg daily. I told her to double up on the Topamax. Maybe, with luck, I could bring this thing under control, but I sure was counting the days until she could get to a psychiatrist because I was over my head in the treatment of acute bipolar mania. I scheduled a return appointment for a week later, and when she didn't show up, I was fearful that something dire had happened.

A couple of days later, I took a call from the psychiatrist. He had admitted her to the hospital. He wanted to inform me of that and to make some inquiries about where we ought to go with therapy. He told me she was quite paranoid and agitated when he saw her, and he chose to discontinue both the Ritalin and the Topamax. He gave her the mood-stabilizer, Abilify, and within twenty-four hours she was much improved, speaking more slowly and without paranoid ideation. She was still having pain, however, and he wondered if resumption of the Topamax would be appropriate. I encouraged him to do that and told him that in the past the drug had been quite helpful to her. It was only because of its appetite-suppressing effect that it was removed. We talked some more, and I told him about her remarkable history of cycling attacks of pain, depression, and catastrophizing each October. I told him I had always wondered why October, and with her description of sexual abuse that month, I understood. Lastly, I asked him if he did not agree that what we had witnessed was bipolar mania. The psychiatrist wouldn't go that far, saying only that she certainly had a "cycling mood disorder" (just as I had written three years before).

I want to mention the reluctance of many psychiatrists to declare a patient bipolar. The diagnosis is stigmatizing and, as we have seen, in the minds of some, shameful. I am sure Lucy's psychiatrist's reluctance with me was an effort to protect his patient from my prejudice (of which there is absolutely none, but there was no way for him to know that). He knew she was bipolar. That is why he used Abilify and why he wanted to resume the Topamax. No harm done. He had treated her very well and got her better quickly. It was a really fine professional performance, and I commended him for that.

Maybe I ought to commend myself also. My writings of a few years before were quite prescient. In a sense, I had actually predicted what was going to happen. Not bad, if I do say so myself. Maybe Lucy's "cycling mood disorder" wasn't really bipolar disease, but it was certainly something like it.

Now back to catastrophizing. It is the vocal expression of obsessive worry. We physicians all recognize it for it is really a rather dramatic clinical display. If I tell a colleague that my patient is catastrophizing, he will know exactly what I am talking about. *The Diagnostic and Statistical Manual* says the phenomenon of catastrophizing, that is excessive worry over a medical condition, is not an obsession. It is something different from OCD. Well, maybe, but if the examples I offer in this book have any meaning, it does seem that catastrophizing travels in company with the bipolar spectrum. Let's look at one more case.

Larissa was fifty years old and afflicted with painful neuropathy. Her peripheral nerves were damaged, cause unknown, and she suffered severe pain in her feet and legs and, to a lesser extent, her hands. My interview was dominated by her incessant vocalization of despair and hopelessness. She kept talking about the bitter pain in her feet, the uselessness of her life, and of her unwanted dependency on her family. Finally, after several minutes of tearful lament, she pressed her palms against her temples as if trying to squeeze her brain and said, "I can't get this pain out of my mind."

Larissa was catastrophizing. Interesting, isn't it that after complaining bitterly of the pain in her feet she offered the declaration that she could not get it out of her mind. She literally could think of nothing else. After her declaration, however, she calmed down a bit, and I was able to take a history.

She was a remarkable woman. She never married and had no need to. Her life was rich enough. She was born of modest means, and she entered the military. There she obtained her RN degree. When her military obligations were completed, she entered the private sector, and within a short order became a charge nurse at a large general hospital and later Director of Nursing. She then elected to abandon that enterprise and enter the field of property management, which she did quite successfully. She had fifty or so employees at the time her illness struck. With that event, she lost everything.

She denied ever having a problem with depression until her pain appeared. To the contrary, she told me through her tears, she was always upbeat and positive—never a down moment. Then the pain struck, and all the good things left. Maybe she had reason to catastrophize.

She was sleepless with the pain, of course, and she freely admitted being depressed for the first time in her life. I couldn't find many clues with Larissa. Her life had been one of achievement. There was no history of childhood abuse, illicit drugs, or any semblance of emotional disorder until she was brought down by pain. I knew I was going to have a difficult problem on my hands. Not to say that Larissa didn't.

I prescribed the usual, Imipramine and Klonopin, and I initiated therapy with Hydrocodone. At the risk of generalization, anticonvulsants can be rather good for nerve pain, and usually the opiates are not. Over the course of several months, I offered her Neurontin, then Lyrica, then Topamax, and then Tegretol. None were in the least helpful. I also prescribed in turn Oxycodone, which failed, and then Morphine, and then Hydromorphone (Dilaudid), one of our strongest opiates. She was insensitive to them all. Few patients have given me the sense of impotency that Larissa did. Usually I can make at least a dent in the suffering. Months into therapy, I had helped her not one bit. On each of her visits, there were tears, frustration, hopelessness, and despair.

"Larissa, we have tried almost everything. There is another drug I use sometimes, though, that I want to try. It is called Methadone, and even though you have failed all of the opiates I have given you, it may just work. Are you willing?"

"Of course," she cried. "I have lost everything, and I want my life back. Let's try something new."

"No promises, Larissa, except that I will leave no stone unturned."

She was a different person when I saw her, for the first time, without tears. She affected comfort and well-being and told me that her pain was almost totally relieved for the first time in two years. Her sleep was restored, and her mind, capable of thinking only of her pain and her hopelessness, was turned off. Remarkably, this effect was achieved with only 15 mg of Methadone—far less than I had prescribed.

Was Larissa bipolar? Certainly not by any of the diagnostic tables. Nonetheless, probably so. The strongest possible evidence for this was her recovery—suddenly and totally not only from pain but from sleeplessness, depression, and obsessive worry. Note that her life before she became ill was one of happiness and unfettered success. She was good at everything she tried to do, and that is a bipolar attribute. Then when she developed the first real illness she had ever known in the form of neuropathy, her pain was severe, and that is also a bipolar attribute. I just happened to hit on Methadone. I chose it not because she was bipolar but because it was something I had not tried before. Nonetheless, looking back on it, I think I cured a victim of the bipolar spectrum and pain with Methadone, and I do believe that excessive worry over a medical condition constitutes an obsession.

I will remind the reader that I have given several examples of patients in whom Methadone (or some other opiate) controlled mood or alleviated depression but did not relieve pain. I wonder if some day I will see something like that in a patient in pain who is catastrophizing. Perhaps an opiate will relieve the catastrophizing but not the pain. I am hopeful that I will see this, and I am certainly going to be looking for it. If I do find it, I will be rather certain that my patient is catastrophizing not because he or she has pain but because he or she has obsessive-compulsive disorder.

CHAPTER 10

Multiple Personalities

Tracy was big, broad-shouldered, and blond. She spoke loudly and rapidly, and she exhibited repetitive facial tics, like grimaces, often accompanied by a barking sound. Tracy clearly suffered, among other things, Tourette's syndrome.

She began the interview by telling me, "My life has been miserable." She developed the tics in her youth and was ostracized for them at home and at school. I asked when the diagnosis of Tourette's was made, and she told me at age twenty-five when she was referred to a university hospital where they took movies of her. Over the years she had been given a vast number of drugs for her Tourette's and her depression. When she came to me she was receiving Lexapro, Klonopin, Seroquel, and Topamax. She also used Imitrex for migraine.

She acknowledged several psychiatric admissions for depression and suicidality and also that a diagnosis of obsessive-compulsive disorder had been made years before. She recalled being depressed as a teenager, and for a long time she took Imipramine. It was the mainstay of her therapy for many years but was ultimately discontinued. She had one son with Tourette's and perhaps obsessive-compulsive disorder whose life as a real estate agent had been rather successful.

Tracy's father died in an automobile accident when she was ten. She had but little memory of that event, but she did spend a lot of time after it with her grandmother who was, she said, a very cold person. In response to my question, she did say that she thought she might have suffered abuse as a child, but she had few memories of her childhood. She had been sleepless throughout her life and developed chronic pain in the form of fibromyalgia eighteen months before coming to me. Her pain was quite periodic with fluctuations in severity. She also suffered mood shifts and did describe intervals of becoming highly "wired."

Tourette's is an uncommon but certainly not rare disease. It almost always begins in childhood. It is characterized by involuntary tics and grimaces and occasionally by head and extremity movements. The tics may be accompanied by barking or yelping sounds, interrupting speech. It is not hard to see why Tracy was ostracized as a child or why her life had been so miserable. Tourette's has a high degree of association with obsessive-compulsive disorder. It certainly was in Tracy. She had the common hand-washing compulsion but also the need to empty her bladder many times each day. Voiding would temporarily relieve her persistent anxiety.

I choose Lithium. There were a couple of reasons, both, I think, pretty good. One was that I suspected underlying bipolarity because of her lifelong depression, her mood lability, her resistance to many forms of treatment, and her chronic pain. I had, even then, long before I discovered the opiate cure, become aware that there was a link between chronic pain and bipolar disorder. Secondly, Lithium was one of the few drugs she had not been exposed to. It was worth a try.

Tracy reported significant improvement on the Lithium. Her moods were more even, and she had even been able to self-arrest some of her attacks of sudden rage. Her facial grimaces and barkings had diminished also. The extent of what I was witnessing, the simultaneous improvement in both bipolarity and Tourette's with Lithium was, I can see clearly now, very slow coming to me. There was really no reason to expect both of them to get better at the same time with one drug. I did not appreciate then that the two disorders might be linked, that they might form a continuum. I added Imipramine, which she had taken with some benefit in the past, and increased the dose of Lithium.

I saw her next, for the first time, in the company of her husband. They were an interesting pair. He appeared to be a rather nonreactive, emotionally lethargic person—the polar opposite of hyperkinetic Tracy. Maybe that was the reason their marriage had endured for some 20 years.

"Dr. Cochran, I wanted Steve to come with me. He has some important things to tell you about me."

"Dr. Cochran, you have really helped Tracy a lot. She is a lot easier to be around. She is not near as nervous as she used to be."

"Is that right, Tracy?"

"Yes, I am a lot better. The pain is better, and I am sleeping well. I want to let Steve talk now."

"Dr. Cochran, every now and then, maybe once a week, Tracy becomes a different person. Her speech changes and she just, well, she just acts different. Something just comes over her, and she becomes a woman I don't know. It is like a trance, I guess, maybe some kind of epileptic convulsion. I don't know much about these things, but something just happens to her. It can last a few minutes but sometimes several hours, and then when she comes to herself, she doesn't remember anything about it. Can you tell me what these things are?"

"Tracy, you are aware that you are having these spells?"

"I don't think so."

"Steve, you say her speech changes. Nonsensical speech? Are the words garbled or slurred?"

"No."

"Can she see and hear and move about with these things?"

"Yes, she is just fine, she can do everything. It is just that she is a different person."

Oh my God, I thought. We've got Tourette's, we've got OCD, we've got bipolarity, chronic pain, and almost certainly multiple personality disorder. I had at that time, and even now, very little experience with MPD although I did know that it is one of the most pharmacy-resistant psychiatric disorders. I confessed to Tracy that I had no real competency in the management of her illness. I told her it was mandatory that she see a psychiatrist. In the meantime, continue the Lithium, Imipramine, Lexapro, Klonopin, Seroquel, and Topamax.

I have already briefly discussed multiple personality disorder, but repetition will do no harm. It is now identified with the perhaps kinder and gentler words, *dissociative identity disorder*. Its victims often give a history of childhood sexual abuse. The disease creates many different people in one. The true personality is periodically arrested and replaced by another, presumably a creation of the subconscious. One of the personalities is often that of a child whose age is that at which sexual abuse first occurred. Usually there are multiple personalities, and the emergence of one or the other probably relates to the type of stressor that precipitates the dissociation.

Tracy, it turned out, had no mental health benefits under her insurance plan. She could not afford psychiatric care. I would just have to do the best I could, acknowledging to her that I was way over my head.

"Nope, you are doing just fine. I really like the Lithium. I don't bark as much as I used to, and my tics are better. My pain is in pretty good control. I am not near as depressed, and I never think of suicide anymore. You are doing a great job. Let's just keep it up."

"Okay, I guess we don't have any other choice. Tracy, let me ask you, do you still have the personality changes? Are you even aware that you do have them?"

"I can't tell for sure, but Steve tells me I am not having as many of them."

Tracy continued to do well on the Lithium and on one of her visits told me that while taking a shower, she suddenly remembered a sexual assault when she was ten years old. This restoration of previously repressed memories appearing under the influence of pharmacy is not rare at all, and I have already given you several examples.

"Tracy, what was your reaction to the memory?"

"I was grateful to remember. It was a missing piece of the puzzle. It doesn't bother me to remember. It helps me to understand."

"I am happy for you. Now, Tracy, we have been almost two years into treatment with the Lithium. Is it still working?"

"Yes. It is not perfect, but it is certainly the best drug I have ever had."

"You are doing so well, I don't think I need to see you for another six months. Come back sooner if there are problems."

There were. She began to develop a tremor, a rapid movement of her fingers and hands. This movement was quite unlike her tic movements. It was incessant, stopping, I was told, only during sleep. I was fearful that her tremor was induced by her Lithium therapy, but I was reluctant to discontinue a drug that had been, however incompletely, beneficial for her. I prescribed the anticonvulsant, Primidone, little used now for epilepsy but a pretty effective drug for the treatment of some tremors. She did not respond, and her tremor was growing ever worse. We had to discontinue the Lithium.

The tremor abated, but depression deepened and with it came mood swings, irritability, and pain. Moreover, her barkings and grimaces reappeared as did her dissociations.

"Tracy, I am over my head in your care. You have a very complex illness, and we have had the good fortune to get a couple of good years out of treatment, but you really need expert psychiatric care. I demand that of you. Whether that is done privately or through a community mental health agency will be up to you. I don't want to abandon you, and I will keep you under my care if you wish, but I absolutely need some help on this. I am not sure which way to go now."

It was three years before I saw her again. Her tics and barkings were worse than they had been when she first came to me.

"I'm back," she grimaced. "My psychiatrist has retired."

"Was he able to help you?"

"Not much. He tried the Lithium again, but the tremors came back. I am still depressed, and I was actually hospitalized a few months ago. I wanted to commit suicide. I am just miserable."

"Did your psychiatrist try different medicines, Tracy?"

"Yes, he tried lots of them, but none of them worked."

"Are you still hurting, Tracy?"

"Yes, worse than ever. I hurt all over my body. The pain keeps me from sleeping."

"Have you ever been given opiates for your pain?"

"No, you never gave me any and none of my other doctors did. They told me I would be an addict if I was given painkillers, and I don't want to be an addict. I have got enough troubles already."

"Tracy, there is an opiate I want to use. It is called Methadone. Have you ever heard of it?"

"Yes, that's what they give heroin addicts, isn't it?"

"Yes, it is used for that, but it is also a good painkiller, and I have learned that it can be mood stabilizing in people with bipolar disorder, and that is what you have. That is why you responded, at least for a while, to the Lithium."

"I know I am bipolar. That is what my psychiatrist said. He also said I had multiple personality disorder, obsessive-compulsive disorder, and Tourette's syndrome just like you did. But Methadone, that scares me."

"It scares lots of people, just like Lithium scares people. Were you frightened of Lithium when I prescribed it six years ago?"

"Yes, I was. Okay, Dr. Cochran, if you think it will help me, I will give it a try."

"Methadone it is. I am writing a prescription. Start at half a pill a day and increase gradually to one three times daily. I will see you in a month. If you have any questions, I want you to call me. I want to stay right on top of this thing."

What an opportunity this was! An opportunity to learn more about Methadone and its effects in mental illness. Perhaps another opportunity for the opiate cure. I had seen it relieve bipolarity, ADD, OCD, PTSD, and even narcolepsy. What would it do for Tourette's syndrome? Could Methadone help when nothing else had? I was engaging in a first order clinical experiment, and I was grateful for the chance. The possibility that Methadone could relieve Tracy's multiple personality disorder did not even enter my mind.

She came back a month later and smiled at me as she spoke. Her words were softer with a slower cadence. "It's magic, Dr. Cochran. There is no other word. It is magic."

"What is better?"

"Everything is better. Absolutely everything."

"Tell me about it. Tell me in detail."

"The pain is gone. It doesn't keep me awake at night. I am not depressed anymore. And my moods aren't shifting. I don't get angry. I am not nervous like I used to be. I am calm. My husband says I am a totally different person. He tells me he likes the new me."

"Keep talking."

"You know, it is really strange. I have always known that I didn't think like other people. I couldn't control my thoughts. But now I think clearly. I comprehend things better. I have even started reading some books. I could never do that before. I remember saying to myself, 'this is the way normal people think.'"

"How about the Tourette's? I haven't seen any tics so far."

"Almost totally gone. Maybe that is the best thing of all. You can't imagine what a relief it is to not be barking at people all the time."

"It is indeed difficult to imagine what that has been like. But we have more things to talk about, haven't we?"

"Yes, we do. My OCD is much better. I don't have to wash my hands, and I don't have to empty my bladder nearly as often, maybe just three or four times a day. I guess that is what normal people do."

"Yes, I suppose that is about average."

"There is something else. Steve wanted me to tell you that I haven't had a single personality change the past month."

"WHAT?"

"Steve says I haven't had a single personality change the past month."

I entered denial.

"Is he sure, really sure? This kind of thing just shouldn't happen. I've never heard of anything like it. It is just can't be."

"It is true, Dr. Cochran."

At the time of this writing we are several months into Tracy's opiate cure. She began to have problems with sweats and sedation from the

Methadone. I changed to Hydrocodone, in the big scheme of things a lesser opiate, but she has blossomed into wellness. The sweats and sedation are gone, and she has obtained relief from the depression, pain, tics, barkings, and personality dissociations. Another cure. Another resurrection. And a question. Is it possible that the opiates, at least one or the other of them, can cure almost anything psychiatric?

Sherry first came to me at her age thirty-seven in 1998. She suffered neck pain and endured a couple of surgical operations without benefit. Her sexual abuse at the hands of her father began at age eleven and continued for several years. She was hospitalized after a suicide attempt in her teens. She experimented for a while with cocaine until she got married at age twenty. It was shortly after that that she started having panic attacks. She began seeing a psychiatrist and was told she had post-traumatic stress disorder and major depression. Over the years she had taken many different antidepressants. Her current treatment was Zoloft and Xanax. Her improvement on those drugs was modest at best. She told me she was sleepless and subject to flashbacks of her abuse. Many of these flashbacks were triggered, she said, by certain smells.

I contacted her psychiatrist and outlined my plan. I did not want to intrude on his therapy, but there were a couple of options that might help our mutual patient. He welcomed my participation.

I gave her Imipramine and Klonopin. She felt well for a couple of days and then sank into a deep depression. I had her terminate the Imipramine, and gave her a kindred drug, Nortriptyline. The same thing happened again. If an antidepressant makes a person more depressed, that is, in my mind, a clue to bipolarity, and I recorded that thought in my note to her psychiatrist. Then I prescribed Ritalin, and she felt that helped not only her depression but to some degree her pain. Sherry has remained on the Ritalin for over a decade, during which time her pain would come and go, and in like manner her depression would come and go. I never knew what to expect when I entered the room to see Sherry. Sometimes she was crying, distraught, and catastrophizing, and other times she was pleasant and engaging, but mostly the former. Cautiously and with some trepidation, I began giving her scant quantities of the opiate, Hydrocodone, to take for her flares. I was a few years away from learning about the opiate cure, but I was rather sure that Sherry was bipolar. When her psychiatrist introduced mood stabilizer therapy, I felt rather sure he did too.

There were intercurrent events. She told me about the trip to Chicago to be with her family. For the first time, at age forty-two, she confronted her father about his abuse of her. Not unexpectedly, she had a terrible flare of pain and depression following the encounter. It lasted for several weeks. On another occasion she told me about a psychiatric hospitalization for depression and suicidal ideation. It was during this confinement that her multiple personality disorder was recognized.

I left her care for that problem in the hands of the psychiatrist who was still prescribing Ritalin among other drugs. I felt my only contribution would be the administration of opiates, an exercise in which I was gradually becoming more competent—and confident. I changed her from Hydrocodone to a stronger opiate, Oxycodone, in an extended release preparation—40 mg every eight hours, not a small dose at all. It did seem to help Sherry's pain. The benefit was incomplete, so I added morphine. She viewed that drug with some favor, and for a couple of years there was some stability in her pain control. Her moods, however, continued to swing.

Satisfied that I was doing as much as I could, I planned to stay the course, and then a problem. One of Sherry's daughters began stealing her medicines. Fearful of telling me about it, Sherry endured several withdrawals and great pain over the course of several weeks. She only told me when she was able to report that her daughter had been admitted to a drug treatment facility. That was a tough time for Sherry, and the interval of depression she experienced with it was quite severe.

The psychiatrist continued his yeoman work, trying one drug after another to control Sherry's moods. I only saw her every three months for prescriptions for her opiates. On one of those occasions, Sherry told me about her other daughter who was seriously ill with bipolar disease. She also suffered frequent migraines and lupus, and she was very much in pain. Sherry wanted to know if I would accept her as a patient. I told her I would if her psychiatrist was agreeable.

Casey was a pitiful being. Her face was puffy and her hair matted with sweat. Her eyes were reddened and tearful. She appeared very anxious, and she was nearly voiceless—whispering words very slowly. Her father gave me the medical history. She had developed migraines at age eighteen, and with one of her attacks actually had a stroke, weakening one leg. Next lupus with joint pain and skin rashes. She became very depressed and was treated with Wellbutrin, a drug that made her manic and suicidal. That is when the diagnosis of bipolar disease was made. Treatment was begun with mood stabilizers and antidepressants. She required large doses, and their effects reduced her to lethargy and torpor, but without them, her father said, she would be very mood unstable and subject to severe panic attacks. She was house-confined and largely bed-confined. She needed assistance with the most fundamental acts of her toilet and hygiene. She was as sick as a young woman can get, and if her disease was not somehow arrested, she surely was going to die from one of the disasters that befall a bed-confined and heavily sedated person, even a young one.

I told Casey and her parents that I would make no intrusion on her psychopharmacy, but that I would prescribe opiates. I started with Hydrocodone, one of the least potent, but I knew where I was going with Casey for I had, in the months preceding, witnessed the opiate cure with Methadone. I didn't think the Hydrocodone would work, and it didn't, so I began Methadone in small doses. Her improvement was not nearly as dramatic as I had seen in others, but it was there. She became more communicative and better groomed. Her emotional angst was clearly abating. I increased the dose over several weeks, and in time her recovery was total. A young woman who but a few months before had been unable to dress herself was riding a bicycle through the neighborhood.

If this story seems familiar to you, it is because I wrote of Casey in *Curing Chronic Pain*. She was one of my first opiate cures.

Surely you know what happened next.

"Dr. Cochran, Casey has done so well on the Methadone. Can we try that drug in me?"

"Probably so. Let's see, you are taking extended release Oxycodone 80 mg every eight hours and extended release Morphine, 30 mg every twelve hours. You have been on that combination several months now. I know we have talked about this before, but I don't recall that you have had any problems with sedation on the drugs."

"No, not at all. They do help my pain somewhat, but not near enough, and they really aren't doing anything for my moods at all. Do you think Methadone could help me like it did Casey?"

"I am willing to prescribe it, Sherry. We will go slowly up to 10 mg every eight hours and let me see you in a couple of weeks."

I don't think I have ever been as confident in the prescription of Methadone as I was with Sherry. Her bipolar daughter had responded to Methadone, and bipolarity is often an inherited disease. That which afflicted Casey almost certainly was afflicting Sherry. The probability of her response was, I thought, quite high, and I had no problem prescribing Methadone on top of her already rather heavy opiate load.

"It is not working, Dr. Cochran. After a couple of days I had severe nausea, and I was very sedated. I had to stop the Methadone. I tried it again later, and the same thing happened. I hate to disappoint you, and I am certainly disappointed myself, but Methadone is not the drug for me. What am I going to do? I really think I may commit suicide. I am never going to have a normal life."

"Sherry, don't do that, and if you feel like you really want to take your life, call Dr. Smith or me right away. Promise me you will do that."

"I will. I promise."

"We are not giving up yet, Sherry. I am disappointed, but there may be a few more rocks to look under."

I had learned that Methadone is not the only opiate that can control bipolarity. It is probably the best opiate for that purpose, but I have seen the same effect with others. Sherry was already on Oxycodone and Morphine, and although they were helping her pain, they were doing very little for her bipolar mood swings. I elected to try Meperidine. It is one of the more troublesome opiates in that it sometimes has an adrenaline-like effect. It can produce convulsive seizures, and, as we have seen, it can interact with some of the antidepressants with fatal consequence. For these reasons, it is infrequently used as ongoing therapy for chronic pain. Nonetheless, I felt it was the way to go. Leave no stone unturned. I gave her a small dose, telling her to ration the pills and use them only when she had a severe siege of pain. If she found them helpful, I would be willing to prescribe them on an ongoing basis.

She told me that the Meperidine didn't do much for her pain, but she had discovered it was the best sleep aid she had ever taken. What a clue! Meperidine was doing something that no other drug had ever done. We were on our way! I wrote a prescription for 50 mg to be taken four times daily.

She returned two weeks later, and I saw right away that we had done it again.

"It is a miracle, Dr. Cochran. It is really working well. It is helping my pain, and my moods are stable. I am not depressed. I am happy. Dr. Smith saw me the other day, and he was thrilled, absolutely astonished."

"I am happy for you, Sherry, I really am. I am a little bit surprised, but I am certainly accepting."

Sherry has been on Meperidine nearly two years now. She has blossomed, at age fifty, into a very engaging woman. She is able to read and enjoy books. Her flashbacks have stopped. She has even coped with the sudden death of her mother without becoming an emotional mudslide, which she had often done under far less provocation in the past. Her life has been totally restored. I enjoy her visits, usually accompanied by her husband, a man I have grown to greatly respect and admire. He had been an exemplary caregiver for his wife and daughter.

No longer faced with this or that crisis, the three of us have time to just chat about Sherry's life, her illness, and her recovery. He tells me that if Sherry misses a single Meperidine pill she becomes quite irritable and, he volunteered, he often has to remind her to take her pills when she gets that way.

"It is the strangest thing, Dr. Cochran. She doesn't have the personality changes anymore."

I hesitated to search my memory for I had forgotten about her multiple personality disorder. When I had first been told about it, I thought it a very important issue but a peripheral one to my treatment. I now know that in the bipolar in pain, nothing is peripheral. There are links, and there is a continuum. I began to appreciate the enormity of what he was telling me.

"WHAT?"

"Dr. Cochran, you have cured her multiple personality disorder. She hasn't dissociated, that's the word, isn't it, in nearly two years."

I was incredulous. "None—no personality changes at all?"

"No, none at all. She used to have them several times a week. I was actually relieved when Dr. Smith made the diagnosis because it gave me some understanding of what was going on. I have tracked this very carefully, and I can tell you that Sherry has eight different personalities. Like many people with MPD, one of her personalities is that of a child. The more common one, though, is an angry, controlling personality. This, I have learned from my research, is the protective personality. When Sherry is threatened, she seeks protection. Sherry goes to the angry personality for refuge."

"I find this all very astonishing. Pain, bipolar disease, post-traumatic stress disorder, and multiple personality disorder all went away with Meperidine. That's what you are telling me, isn't it?"

"Yes, that is what we are telling you," said Sherry.

"And they didn't go away with Morphine and Oxycodone and, if I understand correctly, they didn't go away with any of Dr. Smith's medicines. Is that correct?"

"That is correct. It was the Meperidine. That is what cured her."

"Is Dr. Smith aware that she has recovered from her multiple personality disorder?"

"Yes, he has seen it. He is aware."

"Is he a believer? Does he believe the Meperidine cured the multiple personality disorder?

"He won't talk about it much, but I think he is a believer."

It seems that I make a career out of serendipitous discoveries. I had no anticipation, none at all, that I could actually relieve Tracy's and Sherry's multiple personality disorder by the administration of opiates. Indeed, I had actually disavowed any responsibility for the treatment of that disorder, leaving it in the hands of Sherry's psychiatrist and admonishing Tracy to find one. The reasons for this choice were based on both fear and ignorance. I had actually witnessed a dissociation in one of my prior patients and was quite unnerved by it. It was frightening to witness an able and sentient being become, so completely in voice, manner, and behavior, another person. (I wrote about that experience in *Understanding Chronic Pain*.) I believed (then) that MPD was highly pharmacy resistant and amenable only to counseling, often years of it, not so much to remove the dissociations but to remove the stressors that precipitate them. Bottom line, Tracy and Sherry suffered a hot potato disease, and I didn't want to touch it. I consigned my knowledge of their MPD to the deepest recesses of my memory and, I realized now, did my best to forget about it. How foolish I was! When I ultimately cured them, so unexpectedly, my disbelief was profound. Interestingly, my discovery of the cure was not the result of my inquiries for I had made none. Rather, it was their husbands who informed me of the improbable miracle.

I take pleasure in fanciful thought because sometimes it turns out to be prescient. Let's make a conceptual leap, one that should really not be too hard to do. Let's offer the premise that an efficient and well-functioning opioid system is essential for *emotional* health. This, in the same manner that well-functioning serotonin, noradrenaline, GABA, and dopamine systems are essential for emotional health. We treat their dysfunctions by the administration of pharmacy, which restores the system to vigor. Are we not doing the same thing when we administer opiates and relieve those diseases that I have written about in this and proceeding chapters? Remember, when we administer Prozac to relieve depression, we surmise that we are increasing the quantity or availability of serotonin within the brain. But we don't really know this because we can't measure serotonin levels in the brain. Nor can we measure opioid levels. We don't measure recovery by quantifiable biochemistry, but rather by change in our patient's mood and behavior.

Can we surmise that opioid systems become inefficient in the same manner that the other systems become inefficient? Take a step further. Can we surmise that people develop narcolepsy, attention deficiency, obsessive-compulsive disorder, bipolarity, post-traumatic stress disorder, and even multiple personality disorder *because* their opioid system is either inefficient or overwhelmed?

Now what makes opioid systems inefficient? Probably the same things that make serotonin and all the rest inefficient. Genetics in many cases, but certainly also childhood trauma, including sexual abuse, substance abuse, and cerebral injury.

Fanciful thoughts, perhaps, but not mine alone. Other physicians are beginning to explore, if only in their imagination, the possibility that mental illness is the product of inefficiency of opioid systems within the brain. That theory, tenuous though it may be, would certainly explain the opiate cure.

CHAPTER 11

Cutting and Biting

I have already told you about a couple of bipolars in pain who exercised self-mutilation for the relief of discomfort. Rebecca in the chapter "The Bipolar Way" cut herself to relieve anger and to give her euphoria. Janet, the musician who was so stigmatized by Methadone, cut to relieve anxiety. I will return to her story shortly.

Tim was forty-seven, a big man, over six feet in height and well muscled. He had a ruggedly handsome face but was, nonetheless, one of the more pathetic creatures I had ever seen. He was frequently grimacing in pain. His movements were herky-jerky. His speech also. It was hesitant and grunting in character. He could not articulate a full sentence, only fragments of it. He was restless and quite unable to sustain a single position for more than a few moments, and he had a tremor of his hands and fingers. He appeared anxious and apprehensive, and he was drenched in sweat.

None of his previous physicians, so far as I could tell, had diagnosed his *akathisia*. It is a movement disorder, a form of tremor, and its name derives from the Greek meaning *without sitting* (still). It is a fidgety, ants-in-the-pants tremor that was first described over a hundred years ago. It is often associated with anxiety and is occasionally mistaken for extreme anxiety, and I suppose that is what Tim's physicians attributed his unusual movements to. Akathisia is sometimes seen as part of Parkinson's disease, but the most common cause in our era is as a side effect of drugs, usually the antipsychotics, but also, rarely, the antidepressants.

At age nine, Tim lost a couple of fingers to a radial arm saw. A few weeks later, he witnessed the death of his brother by drowning. He became anxious and was treated with the drug, Limbitrol. It is a combination drug, a mix of Amitriptyline and Librium. It is little used now, but it had its day and was, on occasion, a very effective drug for anxiety and depression. It was in Tim, and he was to remain on it for many years. Could the extended use of Amitriptyline, beginning in the preteen years and extending for a couple of decades, have actually caused his akathisia? It is possible.

He graduated from high school and went to work in a sawmill. He acquired great manual skills and became a competent carpenter, plumber, and electrician. In his early thirties his anxiety and depression escaped control with Limbitrol. For the next fifteen years, at the hands of several doctors, he journeyed through many psychopharmaceuticals. He was told by one of his physicians, a psychiatrist, that he had bipolar disorder. As his depression worsened, he became diffusely painful and was diagnosed with fibromyalgia. It was about that time that his tremors and herky-jerky movements began. At age forty, he developed what was thought to be epilepsy. He would be seized with repetitive muscle jerkings that occurred, almost invariably, just as he dozed off to sleep.

He consulted a neurologist who performed a brainwave test, which was normal. Nonetheless, she treated him, as she certainly should have done, with anticonvulsants. None worked. In the end the neurologist concluded that he did not suffer from a seizure disorder but rather a sleep disorder. And in this judgment I believe she was absolutely correct. Tim had, in spades, a major sleep disorder. He was insomniac, frequently awakening through the night, and he suffered nightmares. His nocturnal muscle jerkings were probably an extravagant display of periodic limb movements. I have written about these before. They are coarse, flailing motions of the extremities that occur during sleep. Tim's seemingly occurred in the hypnagogic interval just as he was going to sleep. Rarely are the movements so repetitive that they could be mistaken for an epileptic convulsion, but I do see how it could happen.

The dutiful neurologist told Tim that she had no more treatment options, but that his movements were not life threatening. She then referred him to a psychiatrist for treatment of his depression and anxiety. After a couple of years of therapy with Zoloft, Klonopin, Zyprexa, and Doxepin in a high dosage of 500 mg nightly, all without restoration of sleep or relief of depression, anxiety, or tremors, he was referred to me for treatment of his chronic pain.

Tim, with his wife, recounted his medical history, telling me that his tremors had become so bad that he could no longer do manual work. He suffered continued anxiety, and he remained quite depressed. I explored the issue of bipolarity and was told that Tim didn't have the expected ups and downs, and that he was actually quite easy to be around. There were no problems with irritability or anger, just anxiety, depression, shakes, and increasingly frequent drenching sweats.

Let's see where I stood as I began Tim's treatment. He clearly had the tremor, akathisia, and also depression, anxiety, and chronic pain. Was he bipolar? He certainly lacked the classic mood swings although, as I have suggested before, ongoing and treatment-resistant depression and chronic pain can certainly be symptoms of that disorder. Moreover, he suffered narcoleptic nightmares in the form of hypnagogic hallucinations. And the sweats? Where do they fit in? Recall the story of the young bipolar from New Hampshire who told me that his manic spells made him feel "hot, sweaty, and nervous."

What to do? I knew I would be scraping the bottom of the pharmaceutical barrel because there were not many drugs left that he had not taken. He was already on Hydrocodone for pain. I added Oxycodone. I then began my foray into mind drugs. I gave him Seroquel without benefit and then Ritalin with the same result. I tried Clonidine, a blood pressure medicine, that can help people with attention deficit disorder, and maybe Tim had a bit of that. Then Primidone, occasionally useful for tremors. Next Triavil, a combination of Amitriptyline and the antipsychotic, Trilafon. It was widely used in years past but almost never now because of its capacity to produce a tremor known as *dyskinesia* (more later). It did no good but thankfully made his akathisia no worse. Next Propranolol, a blood pressure drug that sometimes helps anxiety. I even tried Strattera. I was getting nowhere. There was nothing to do but slowly increase the Oxycodone dosage. At that time I was more fearful of opiate therapy than I am now, but he was getting some pain relief. I never anticipated, however, that his sweats, tremors, anxiety, and depression would all go away when we reached the necessary threshold of dosage of that drug.

We were some four years into treatment, and Tim was taking 180 mg of extended release Oxycodone every eight hours. Quite a big dose but by no means remarkably effective. I did, however, in one of my office notes at that time record that he was somehow looking better. I couldn't articulate it very well, but there was just a sense that he had improved, and also that I had no real idea as to why for I had made no significant alterations in his therapy over the course of several months. Shortly after that note was written, I first witnessed the opiate cure. I elected to do the obvious, adding Methadone, the miracle opiate.

Tim returned to tell me, in the company of his wife, that he simply couldn't take the medicine. He said it made his skin crawl, nauseated him, and gave him headaches. I agreed that we had to discontinue the drug, but, and I remember this well, Tim had a look about him that I had not seen before. He wasn't sweating. His tremors and jerks had diminished. His speech was better articulated, and there was just an air of calmness that I had not witnessed before. His wife agreed.

I offered morphine, and that went nowhere. Then an event. Tim had begun to do some carpentry work around his house, an activity impossible when he first came to see me. He struck his hand with a hammer, and the pain was excruciating. With it came a return of his total body pain and the reappearance of sweats and jerking. When he told me about it, he said the only way he could get pain relief was to bite himself. He then pulled down his lower lip so I could see the mucosal surface, and it was a mass of bloody, macerated tissue.

"We have never talked about this, Doc, but the only way I can get relief of pain is to injure myself. A lot of times in the past I had to cut or bite myself to make pain go away. I found the quickest and easiest way to do it is to just hold my lower lip between my teeth and bite it hard."

"Tim, I don't know much else to do but give you more Oxycodone. I am a little bit fearful because you are taking a very big dose. Are you having any trouble with it at all—sedation or shortness of breath?"

"None of that at all, and I have to tell you, of all the drugs I have taken, Oxycodone is the only one that ever helped me at all."

"Okay, you can go up to 240 mg every eight hours. Call me if you have problems and get back to see me in two weeks."

It was just about the highest dose of Oxycodone I had ever given anybody, but I felt that I could not deny him the only drug that helped him, however incompletely.

He was a different man—calm, smiling, moving gracefully without tremors, and he was no longer sweating or biting. He offered me a view of his lower lip, and it had returned to normal. He told me was back at work at the sawmill.

We had finally reached, after years of my opiate fearful hesitancy, the right dose of the right drug. And this applies to the treatment of both pain and the bipolar spectrum. Seven hundred and twenty milligrams per day of Oxycodone was Tim's threshold. It was far beyond the FDA-recommended maximum dosage of the drug.

The transformation that has come to him is, frankly, unbelievable. Formerly tremulous, sweaty, anxious, depressed, and impaired in his ability to articulate speech, he now delighted me with his little jokes.

"Doc, have you heard about the man who went to the psychiatrist?"

"No, Tim, tell me about the man who went to the psychiatrist."

"He told the doctor he was having dreams at night. All he would dream of was teepees and wigwams—that's all, just teepees and wigwams."

"And?"

"The doctor told him he was too tense."

"Pretty good, Tim, pretty good."

Tim had become charming, gifted in conversation, and witty (the bipolar way?). He was contentedly happy, and I think my therapy may have made him just a little bit manic because he has gone out and bought a forklift. He planned to build a new sawmill, his very own.

Then a bump in the road, a big bump. His pain, sweats, tremors and herky-jerky movements all came back. He once again exposed his lower lip, and it looked like hamburger meat. What had gone wrong?

It didn't take me long to figure it out. I had been giving Tim an extended release preparation of Oxycodone. That particular drug is widely known by the brand name, Oxycontin. It comes in some very high dosages and is therefore one of the more popular preparations for the drug abuser. It can be injected, snorted, or inhaled if the material is burned. The manufacturers, in a laudable attempt to forestall abuse of their drug, reformulated it with a tamper-proof matrix. There is no doubt in my mind that the new Oxycontin is less effective milligram for milligram than the original product. I suspect that its tamper-proofness impairs its absorption. I have addressed this problem in several patients by increasing the dose of Oxycontin or, in some cases, adding immediate release Oxycodone (which is not tamper-proof). Tim was already on as much immediate release Oxycodone as he could tolerate because of nausea, so I had no recourse but to increase the Oxycontin from 240 to 300 mg every eight hours. Nearly a gram of the stuff, an outrageous dose, but I had to do it.

Tim got better. The sweats, the tremors, and the pain were improved, and he no longer had to bite himself. He had by no means returned to his witty jocularity, but he certainly is not as depressed as he had been. Discouraged would be a better word.

"I never should have bought that forklift. I'll never be able to work again."

"Don't give up yet Tim. I will go up on the dose of Oxycontin even more if I have to, but first I want you to try the Methadone again. I know you had trouble with it before, but a lot of people tolerate it and get relief when they try it a second time. It is worth a try."

I knew I could get Tim better. It was going to take a lot of medicine, but I was sure I could do it. But there was trouble on the horizon. I received a phone call from Tim's insurer's pharmacy service. I was challenged about the high dosages of Oxycontin. I did the best I could for Tim, but very few doctors and pharmacists are really aware of the opiate cure and the sometimes high doses necessary to achieve it. I did tell the pharmacist that Tim's akathisia had been relieved as well as his pain and depression. The pharmacist was rather generous with me, far more than I expected. He told me he would approve sixty days of this dosage and then a reappraisal. He did express to me that he was sure I was using the Methadone in order to get him on a lower dose of Oxycodone. I tried to tell him as nicely as I could that I wasn't trying to get Tim off anything. I was trying to get Tim well.

And I did. Tim was smiling broadly when he came back to see me. He told me he was back on the Methadone, taking one pill each night, and that he was sleeping better. His pain was diminished, and he was making plans again to build his own sawmill. We had a nice visit, and at the conclusion he asked me if I had time for a joke.

"Sure."

"Have you heard about the two cannibals eating a comedian?"

"Two cannibals eating a comedian, is that what you said?"

"Yeah, Doc. One of them said this meat tastes kinda funny."

A word now about the extraordinarily high doses of opiate that Tim required for his care. It is now well recognized that there are several variants of opiate receptors, and which of these an individual possesses is probably genetically endowed. Thus, one person's opiate receptor may be extremely sensitive, and that person will respond to low dosage opiate therapy. In others, the receptor is highly insensitive and will respond only to extremely high doses. We also know that there is great variation in the enzyme systems that metabolize the opiates (and virtually all other drugs), that is, degrades them from a biologically active chemical to an inactive one. To complicate matters further, the function of the enzyme systems can be influenced by other medications the patient is taking. It is good to be reminded that our medicines are highly standardized, but we humans who take them are not. Thus, the great variation in drug dosages needed to achieve the desired effect.

Tim's akathisia went away totally with Oxycodone. The tremor-relieving effect of opiates is not rare. They are indicated, off label, for the treatment of restless legs. I have a painful patient with severe and treatment-resistant *essential tremor*, a rapid to and fro movement of the fingers and hands. To the surprise and delight of her neurologist, it went away when I prescribed Oxycodone. Another patient with chronic wrist pain following a fracture developed over the course of several years a *choreoathetoic* tremor in that extremity. It is a writhing, twisting, serpentine kind of movement, and hers was quite severe, involving most of the right arm. Her tremor was probably a reflection of the *centralization* of pain. Stated in the most general terms, it means that when pain becomes an established part of brain function, it alters other parts. A tremor in a painful extremity is by no means rare although I had never seen one so severe as hers. She was elderly and none of her doctors had any interest in giving her opiates for her pain and thus to me. I prescribed Oxycodone, and within a couple of days her tremor stopped completely. It has not recurred the six years she has been under my observation.

Where does Tim's akathisia stand in relation to his pain, depression, and all the rest? It went away along with all the rest with Oxycodone and later Methadone. Does that make akathisia part of the bipolar spectrum? I suspect so, for I have learned in the treatment of those in pain that no symptom is peripheral, that no symptom is unimportant. It is all one disease, one very big disease.

Neil was twenty-eight when he first came to me, recently married with three stepchildren. Some eight years before, he suffered a compound fracture of his right forearm. He required surgery with the insertion of metal plates and screws. He was back at work in the landscaping business some eight weeks later. His forearm remained somewhat painful, but he controlled it with over-the-counter analgesics. Some six months before coming to me, he fell from a height and landed on his extended right arm. There was no fracture and no evidence of damage to the muscles or nerves, but his pain became much worse, and he developed "electricity feelings" in his right arm. Since his fall, his pain had become climate-sensitive, worsening in cold and wet weather. He had become sleep-impaired, subject to vivid dreams, and also for the first time, depressed.

I have written in earlier books and a bit in this one about the experience of remembered pain. Neil had a severe injury to his forearm years before coming to me. He had gotten by just fine using drugs like Ibuprofen. Then another injury to the same extremity, much less severe than the first, at least by our measure of testing, but this time his pain was severe. It was perhaps a case of a new pain bringing an old pain along for the ride. Pain, which had been in control before, was out of control under the sponsorship of a new injury. It happens a lot.

He offered a past history of a very unhappy childhood, watching his father repeatedly beat his mom, this until they divorced at his age thirteen. As a youngster he was diagnosed with attention deficit disorder and treated for a while with Ritalin. He acknowledged learning problems in school and also trouble with the law. He went to jail at age eighteen for possession of stolen goods. He told me he took anger management courses while in jail. He was taking Oxycodone provided by his primary care doctor. I continued it and prescribed Ritalin.

When he came back he told me with excitement that he had noticed tremendous improvement in mental focus and attention, and that he hadn't snapped at anybody for the two weeks he had been on it. The Oxycodone was not doing a very good job of controlling his pain, however, and he told me for the first time that when his pain was severe, he could bite his lower lip and make the pain go away. At my request he pulled his lip down, and it looked just like Tim's, hamburger meat.

"Neil, do you get any kind of rush out of biting yourself? Do you feel euphoric or does it make your mood better?"

"No, it just makes the pain go away. That is all it does."

I added Methadone, but he tolerated it poorly because of nausea. I increased the dosage of both Oxycodone and Ritalin. He told me it was "a good combo." Then another trauma. A tree had fallen on his roof during a storm, and in his efforts to remove it, a large limb fell against his right forearm. He had to start chewing his lip again. With time his pain diminished, and he quit biting. He finally connected with a psychiatrist, as I had advised him some months before. The diagnosis was bipolar disorder, and the psychiatrist prescribed Lithium. I was pleased to have the psychiatrist on board, and I thought our therapy with Oxycodone, Ritalin, and Lithium could control both his mood and pain.

It was not to be. I don't know what the provocation was, but Neil became enraged at his psychiatrist and left his care. He sent me a fax saying he was going to stop all of his medicines. The bipolar way again. I called him and found him in an angry mood. He told he was having a lot more arm pain, and he was biting his lip again. I had him come into my office.

"Neil, I don't know what upset you with the psychiatrist. He was only trying to help you. I sure don't want you to stop your medicines."

"They are not helping me anymore. I want to be rid of them."

"Neil, I want to talk to you a little bit about bipolar disease. You have it, and that is why you have so much pain. You are subject to impulse and recklessness, and you have got to learn to control that and your anger. I will do what I can, but you have to do some of the work."

"Okay, Doc. I'll do what you tell me, but my pain is bad, and the drugs aren't working. What are we going to do?"

I wrote him a prescription for Lamictal and told him to return in two weeks.

"I love that drug, Doc! It makes me feel good. I wake up happy every day. That has never happened before."

"That's good, Neil. The effect you have experienced is not uncommon."

Sometimes I think that accident-proneness is a symptom of bipolarity. Neil had already had three of them—all damaging the right forearm. Such is the lot of the bipolar. They seem to have very bad luck. Some of the time, to be sure, it is of their own making, but others, perhaps not.

It was within a month of starting his Lamictal that Neil lacerated his right hand, the right again, at work. There was extensive damage to tendons and nerves. Surgery was required, and the pain was intense. When I saw him first after his surgery, he told me that his emotions were in good shape, but that his pain was horrible. He had to bite his lip again, and he pulled it down to show me—red, swollen, and bloody. I increased the Oxycodone, and he gradually got better.

A year into his care, he was really doing rather well until he experienced yet another injury. He sprained his back lifting a heavy bag of material. I didn't think it was a major injury, but I gave him a few days of an anti-inflammatory drug and a prescription for Meperidine tablets to carry him through the pain because the Oxycodone was not touching it.

Neil offers an interesting study in the behavior of pain along the dimension of time. His second forearm injury, much less severe than the first, was excruciatingly painful, probably because of the first. It was a new pain bringing an old pain along for the ride. And then he discovered that a new pain (biting) could relieve an old pain (forearm). And then a new pain (back sprain) was totally unrelieved by drugs that had been controlling his old pain (forearm).

Neil returned in just a few days to tell me that his back pain was totally relieved by the Meperidine and the effect he got from it was exactly the same as he had experienced when he bit his lip. No other painkiller, he told me, had ever done anything like that.

A *counterstimulus* often relieves pain. We bump our knee, and we rub it to create a different sensation to override the pain. This is the same effect that is achieved with the widely used Transcutaneous Electrical Nerve Stimulation (TENS) unit. This creates a buzzing or electric sensation that overrides a deeper and more severe pain. We achieve the same effect when we tie a band around our head to relieve a migraine or place an ice pack for the same purpose. Pain is diminished by a lesser sensation, but biting one's lip, a very sensitive area, is not exactly another sensation. But both Tim and Neil told me it made the pain go away—at least for a while. It didn't diminish it. It made it go way. And that effect, at least in Neil, was exactly duplicated by the opiate, Meperidine. Remarkable stuff, and I can't begin to tell you that I understand it.

Priscilla found out about me on the Internet and sent me this e-mail:

> Dear Dr. Cochran:
> I have been in terrible pain for so long. A lot of people don't believe in chronic pain. "It's all in your head." Well, in my case a lot of it is in my head. I have had so much bottled up inside me for so many years, I can't remember the last time I slept for more than two hours. I have been angry for so long, and I don't even know why. My mind feels horrible. I talk in circles all the time, and I talk so fast a lot of people can't understand me. I have cut off ALL my friends. The only people I talk to are my mom, husband, daughter, and son-in-law. I can go from good mood to evil mood in 1.0 second. I am not talking about a little angry; I am talking about evil moods—moods that frighten me. My mind races even when I am trying to sleep. I can't concentrate anymore at all. I have seen a zillion doctors and four shrinks. They couldn't help me. Most said I was mildly depressed. Mildly depressed my bottom. Let's see—self-mutilating, angry for no reason, suicidal, racing thoughts spinning out of control, and my pain level is a 12 on a scale of 1 to 10. A zillion doctors and four shrinks seem to think I am okay. What is wrong with this picture?

Suicidal thoughts, self-mutilating, mood swings—angry, evil moods that would make Linda Blair in the *Exorcist* look like Little Miss Sunshine. On top of that, I am in excruciating pain 24/7.

I guess I need to tell you a little bit about me. I was brutally raped by a physician when I was 35. Within a short while after that, I was in a horrible boating accident with my daughter. She was the only one not injured (I thank the Lord above for that). I had bones shattered, disks ruptured, you name it in my back, arms, and neck.

I tried for ten years to avoid surgery. I finally gave in in 1999. I had a spinal fusion and in less than a year it had to be redone twice.

I applied for Social Security Benefits over 18 months ago, and my attorney said even if I got it, it would be 12 months or so before receiving benefits. I was once a Type A personality plus. I didn't have an off button. I was always in first gear going 24/7, goal oriented, and very proud of my success. Now I am depressed, helpless, and dependent.

I have read your book, and I know you can help me.

Sincerely,

Priscilla Jones

"Priscilla, your e-mail is quite good. It really gives me a lot of information, but we do have a lot more to talk about."

"Thank you. After reading your book, I knew you would be interested in more things than just my pain."

"Well, again, you did a good job. Let's see, you have seen many doctors including four psychiatrists. Have any of them suggested that you might have bipolar disorder or maybe attention deficit disorder?"

"No. Like I wrote you, they say I am 'mildly depressed.'"

"What medicines are you taking now?"

"I am taking Hydrocodone and Methadone from a pain clinic that is nothing but a drive-through pharmacy. I am also taking Xanax and Cymbalta from a mental health clinic."

"Are they helping you?"

"A little, at least the pain meds and the Xanax do. Cymbalta hasn't done anything yet."

"Did the Methadone help your moods in any way? Did it make you feel calm?"

"No, nothing has ever helped my moods except cutting."

"Well, we were going to get to that sooner or later, so tell me about it."

"It began about a year ago. I was feeling so bad I was actually suicidal. I just had this enormous evil anger in me, and I read about people who mutilate themselves to get rid of bad thoughts. So I began cutting myself with razor blades. It really worked. It worked for several hours. It is hard to describe. It was almost a euphoria. It was instant relief and gratification."

"How often do you do it?"

"Whenever I am really stressed."

"Once a week? Once a month?"

"Probably, on average, two times a month. It has been about six weeks since I last did it, and I think that is because I made an appointment with you. Your writings have made me very hopeful, and I pray that you don't retire before you get me figured out."

"I don't plan to."

Priscilla's was a life of enthusiasm and achievement, then a sexual assault, and within but a few weeks a major accident with multiple fractures and several ruptured discs in her back. That is when the depression kicked in and with time, her evolution into bipolar disorder. I was interested in the fact that the Methadone, at a dosage of 20 mg three times daily, did nothing to stabilize her moods. Methadone failures are usually due to intolerance to the drug—nausea, sedation, whatever. If the bipolar can tolerate the drug, it usually is pretty helpful, but there are always exceptions. That said, I was sure Priscilla was bipolar and with it attention deficient. ("My mind races.") I told her to continue taking the medicine she was currently taking, and I added Klonopin and Ritalin.

She reported that the mood swings were not as bad, and that she could think better. Her thought-racing had largely gone away. I added Lamictal as a mood stabilizer, and over the next several weeks she did well. She emphasized on each return visit that she was not cutting herself. Then an intercurrent event—unfortunately a common one in the lives of those in pain. Her mother discovered how many different medicines she was taking and, alarmed by the number, threw them all away. Priscilla was two weeks without her medicines before coming back to me.

"I feel just terrible. My moods are shifting, and it is very queer, I don't want to eat. I have no desire for food at all. Am I trying to kill myself?"

"I don't know, Priscilla, I really don't know. Let me ask you this. Did you start cutting yourself when that happened?"

"No, I wanted to, but I resisted it. Aren't you proud of me?"

A pattern was emerging. Priscilla was not measuring her improvement in terms of pain, depression, anger, or mood swings. Clearly, her most important measurement was her ability to refrain from cutting herself.

Whether her emotional swings related to the trauma of her encounter with her mother or were due to the absence of two weeks of bipolar medicine, I didn't know, but I resumed her prior therapy and encouraged consultation with a psychiatrist. I told her I would help her find one who would recognize and treat her bipolar disorder. Priscilla told me she had no interest in ever seeing a psychiatrist again.

A few months later, she returned for a routine appointment and began conversation by saying, "I am cutting again."

"Why, Priscilla? Is there some stressor that is making you do this?"

"Yes, you are my stressor. I am so afraid and anxious that you are going to retire, and I won't have you. You are my crutch."

I increased the Lamictal dosage.

I saw her a month later. She told me with enthusiasm that she had done no cutting at all. She had discontinued the Lamictal because it was too expensive, and she didn't think it was helping. On our next encounter, she told me that her moods were in good shape, that she wasn't cutting, and she would like to try another pain drug, Oxycodone. I told her that that was not an unreasonable request, but how did she know about that drug?

"My son-in-law shared some of his Oxycodone with me, and it has been the best pain drug I have ever had."

"Did it help your pain and your mood or just the pain?"

"I think it helped both."

"Priscilla, I am giving you Oxycodone 15 mg three times daily."

I then performed the physician's necessary obligation and reminded her that she really shouldn't be using other people's medicines. I acknowledged, however, to myself—not to Priscilla—that many people that I attend and write about find the right drug, the drug that ultimately cures because they used somebody else's medicine. I wonder if we physicians could diminish that activity by being imaginative and aggressive in our treatments. Why couldn't we find the right drug instead of making the patient find it? The opiate cure has taught me, and I have certainly tried to send this message in this book, that there almost always is a drug out there for everybody. It is the physician's job to find it, not the patient's.

The Oxycodone was a pretty good mood stabilizer for Priscilla. When she told me this, she also told me that she had gone through her disability hearing and, with pride, that she didn't cut even though the experience was very stressful to her. Let's read about it in her own words.

Dear Dr. Cochran:

I had to go to court a while back, and this was not a friendly environment for me. Shortly before my court date I started panicking. I knew I would need my razors, Band-Aids, peroxide, needle, and thread—all my equipment for cutting. I keep it in a small green box. It was with me at all times. Big problem—can't take razors into a courthouse. If the outcome was not the one I wanted, I knew I couldn't make it home before I cut. I am so like a junkie. The junkie has to know where his next fix is coming from. I have to make plans whenever I leave the house to be sure I have my cutting supplies at all times. For the first time in so so long, I didn't take my cutting supplies. This was a huge step, but when I got to the courtroom, I wanted my husband to go pick up some razors at the drug store in case I needed to cut myself.

I was before the judge for hours. For the first time in so long, I DIDN'T CUT. I am on the right road now. It is still a very bumpy road. At this point my roads aren't like everyone else's roads. All roads have curves, hills, up, and downs. Maybe I always get the wrong directions because my hills are like Mt. Everest. My downs are like a bad stock market. My curves are like the biggest rollercoaster in Florida.

Priscilla Jones

Priscilla and I have been together now over two years. Hers was not a lightswitch, sky-is-blue-again recovery. It was slow, but she is now a different person. The anger, so evident in her first e-mail to me, has gone away. There is a calmness and confidence and control about her that is far removed from her behaviors when I first saw her. She tells me that the very thought of cutting herself makes her viscerally ill, nauseous, and sweaty. I told her I thought that was a good sign.

The people I have described in this chapter were bipolar. All obtained relief from anxiety or pain with self-mutilation. I really don't know whether this exercise occurs exclusively in bipolars or not, but I do wonder.

I also wonder about that art form known as the tattoo. I think I see more tattoos in bipolars than in others, but I really can't be sure, and I can certainly offer no statistical analysis. Nonetheless, I had an interesting idea, and I elected to pursue it.

Joe first came to see me at age thirty-two with a history of chronic back pain. He offered an extraordinary family history of depression and acknowledged also depressed mood throughout his life. He experienced some suicidal ideation along the way but no attempt. He came to a lumbar fusion some four years before. He also about that time was started on Prozac on which drug he remained. He acknowledged a real problem in the past with disinhibited spending, sufficiently severe for him to turn all financial affairs over to his wife. He had extensive and colorful tattoos over his arms and neck.

I started him on Methadone and then Lithium. He did rather well. I told him that he did suffer bipolar disorder. He told me that he was happy to know it. It explained a lot of his problems. We have had a very nice relationship. There have been issues, however, and recently he had developed more mood shifting. I increased the Methadone dosage and advised him that it was time to get a psychiatrist on board. He was quite comfortable with that notion, and he thanked me for the care I had been giving him the past three years.

"Joe, if you don't mind, I would like to ask you some questions. They may be personal, and if they offend, you can tell me so."

"I'll tell you anything you want to know."

"About your tattoos. I see you have them over your arms and some on your neck. I don't know if you have them on your torso or legs, but you do have some pretty impressive tattoos. Could I ask you why you get them?"

"Of course. I look at it that way, it's an adornment. I am proud of the appearance of my tattoos. There is another issue, though. I am not a very handsome man. I am obese. I feel like my tattoos take people's attention away from my face and body, and I kind of like that."

"I understand it is quite painful to be tattooed. Is that correct?"

"Yes, most people say it is very painful."

"And you?"

He laughed and said, "Oh, it is an endorphin high like you can't imagine. It is the most wonderful feeling in the world, and it may last for days after the tattoo is done."

Now let's go back to Janet, the Methadone-fearful young musician from the chapter "Cure and Stigma." As I was reviewing her chart for her story to be included in this book, I realized that she was quite a bit late for a return appointment, and I worried about her. I wondered if she had removed herself from the stigmatizing Methadone and left me. I was pleased when she finally returned. I returned to the issue that had so bothered her.

"Are you still taking the Methadone?"

"Yes."

"Still doing good?"

"Pretty good."

"Are you still ashamed of taking Methadone, Janet?"

"Yes, I am afraid I am. I just can't get over it. I don't let anybody know about it. None of my friends know. Nobody except my father. He tells me it has been a lifesaver for me. He wants me to continue it."

"It is your choice, Janet. You know that. Let me tell you something. There is not much recognition out there now that drugs like Methadone can help bipolar disease, but there is a lot more than there was just three or four years ago. The idea is catching on, and I think in four or five years it will probably come into general knowledge, and you won't have to be ashamed of taking a drug that is curing you."

Her eyes moistened, and she said, "Thank you, you cannot believe how much comfort that gives me."

"Need more Methadone now?"

"Yes. I am out of it now."

"You should have been out of it weeks ago, Janet. What is going on?"

"I reduced it. You had me taking six pills three times daily, but I am now taking three."

"And what is happening?"

"I am getting more depressed. The migraines are coming back. My fibromyalgia is bothering me."

"Janet, that is almost certainly because you have reduced the Methadone. I think we can relieve your symptoms if we get back to the original dose."

"I am willing. I just had to do this. I had to see if I could go without the Methadone. I realize now I can't."

"Janet, I am writing another book, and I am going to put you in it. You are an example of one stigmatized by taking opiates. But there is another chapter in there on self-injury. I have reviewed your chart and am aware that you cut yourself to get relief from anxiety. Is that correct?"

"Well, I wasn't a cutter."

"But you said you cut."

"A cutter does it by ritual. I just did it when I was anxious, when I was really panicky."

"Did it relieve your anxiety?"

"Yes, but it is very curious. I only cut when I had a panic attack. When I cut I quit panicking. I don't know if the cutting was part of the panic or if it was something I did to relieve the panic. Do you understand what I am talking about?"

"That is very insightful, Janet. You are not sure whether your anxiety made you cut or whether you cut to relieve anxiety. It is a good question, and I don't have an answer, but let me compliment you. You expressed that very well. Janet, let me ask you, where did you cut?"

"My thighs and my wrist and forearm. Here, let me show you something."

She pulled up her long-sleeved sweater, exposing the left forearm and a rectangular tattoo about two inches wide and five inches long. It was a monochromatic maroon, and it featured no ornamentation at all other than a thin crescent of pale, unadorned flesh. It was neither colorful nor artistic, but I made no comment about that, of course.

"I got the tattoo to cover up my scars. Look, you can't see them at all."

"That is interesting. Your tattoo is on your left arm. Do you have one on the right?"

"No, because I cut with my right hand."

"Makes sense."

We had a nice visit, and we said our goodbyes, it suddenly occurred to me to ask one more question.

"Janet, I am told that getting tattooed can be extremely painful. Did you experience a lot of pain when you had it done?"

"No, it was the most euphoric experience I have ever known. It took four and a half hours to get the tattoo, and I was happier then than I had ever been in my life. It lasted into the next day."

"Thanks for sharing that with me."

What does it all mean? Somehow my sense is that it is not unimportant. I am making more inquiries of my tattooed patients. I had avoided doing that for fear of hurting feelings or being too intrusive. I don't know why I should really worry about that because I am already very intrusive in my questionings.

Most patients react favorably to my inquiry. They want to tell me about their experience with tattooing. And yes, I am finding other bipolars who get a euphoric rush to the extent that they greatly anticipate getting a tattoo. One woman told me the feeling is exactly the same as the feeling she derives from a shopping spree. Most tell me that tattooing is a very addictive experience.

There are, as I have already indicated, a lot of dots to connect, and tattooing, believe it or not, is one of those dots. It is not unimportant, just as nocturnal voidings, in medical parlance, nocturia, is also not unimportant.

CHAPTER 12

Voiding

Dear Dr. Cochran:

I am a 28-year-old female with a rare congenital defect. I was born with Sprengel's Deformity and went undiagnosed until I was about 21 years old. My right shoulder blade sits high on my back and neck and is misshaped. The rhomboid muscle on the right side is atrophied and pretty much nonexistent. I have been told that what used to be my rhomboid has been replaced with scar tissue and basically glues my shoulder blade in place. My sixth cervical vertebra is turned sideways, facing the right, and is possibly connected to my shoulder blade by some type of connective tissue. There is very little information available on Sprengel's, but I have done a lot of reading over the years in hope of finding help. Unfortunately for me, most people with Sprengel's are diagnosed very early in life and are only surgical candidates before age six or so. I cannot even begin to count how many doctors I have seen over the years looking for anyone who could offer me hope. However, every road for me has been a dead end. Orthopedic surgeons turn me away because I am not a surgical candidate. Anesthesiologists have performed cortisone injections in my neck with no relief. Additionally, I have been told by anesthesiologists that pain blocks are not going to work for me due to my structural defects. I feel as though I have nowhere to turn, and no one can help me. I am in constant pain in my neck and my upper back. I am used to compensating for my "weak" right arm and back, but the pain has been pretty tough to deal with. I consider myself to have a very high tolerance for pain. I am pretty good throughout the morning, but as the day goes on it gets much worse. I recently read that the weight of the arm is responsible for a lot of the pain with Sprengel's, and I have to agree with that. Around 4:00 p.m. every day is when my pain really starts getting tough. If I take something for it and don't let the pain get out of control, I can deal with it pretty well and am highly functional. However, if I don't treat it before it gets bad, it makes for a pretty bad evening and night. As long as I go to bed pain free, I am able to sleep fairly well and wake up feeling pretty good the next day.

I have been told quite a few things about my pain. Most doctors tell me that I am too young to be in pain, and I am too young to take medicine for it. I am told a lot that I need to accept it and learn to live with it. I have been told that I need to exercise more, and that would help me. I have been told that I need to see a psychiatrist to help me cope with my pain. I have been refused medication for my condition because I am told that I may become addicted. All of this has been extremely frustrating to me. When my shoulder is bothering me, I am unable to do much of anything other than lie in bed or sit on a couch protecting my arm and neck. I am a very active person with two small children, so you can only imagine how aggravating that is. All I really want is to be able to live my life with my husband and kids with less pain. Please consider accepting me as your patient.

Sincerely,

Lori Johnson, RN

She was a stunningly attractive brunette, a nurse, working in a community hospital. Interestingly, she had been a college softball player and had been unimpaired by her deformity until about six years before she came to me. It was about this time that, recently married, she suffered several miscarriages and entered a depression that was benefited by Zoloft. She ultimately carried two pregnancies to term and experienced, on both occasions, postpartum depression lasting a couple of months. She denied any real problem with mood shifts but did say that she has "occasional dark feelings." Her sleep was frequently interrupted by pain.

She told me that she feels her doctors view her as a drug-seeker. One in particular laughed at her when she told him she had Sprengel's Deformity. He said he had never heard of such a thing, and that she came to see him only to get drugs. She did occasionally get Hydrocodone in limited quantities from doctors or walk-in clinics. That was the only drug that gave her any relief from her afternoon pains. She hoarded the pills and only used them when the pain was at its worst—maybe a couple of times a week.

This hoarding of drugs is a very common behavior, and it is identified as *pseudoaddiction*. The person is not an addict but is simply trying to protect him or herself from pain. No one, it seemed, was willing to do that for her.

"Lori, I will give you the Hydrocodone. You need it, and you are worthy of it, and I don't want you to be ashamed of taking it."

I continued my inquiries and concluded by asking if she ever suffered distressing, realistic dreams.

"Why yes. I have them all the time. I have had them for years."

"Do you ever have the sense that you are paralyzed, that you can't move when you wake up?"

"Yes, that happens most every time."

"Do you get sleepy during the day?"

"A little, maybe, but not bad."

"Do you ever have sudden falls where your legs give out with you?"

"I don't think so, but something I have noticed is that I have become very clumsy. I have really lost a lot of control in my hands. Things will just fall out of them for no reason. Is that important?"

"Probably. Lori, these dreams and paralysis are features of narcolepsy, and I think that may give us a real clue on how to treat you. I am starting you on a stimulant drug. I am sure you have heard of it. It is called Adderall."

"Yes, that is what they give kids with ADHD, isn't it?"

"Yes, but I am not giving it to you for that. You told me that your mental focus and memory were good, didn't you?"

"Yes."

It was to be yet another miracle. She was smiling and very excited. She told me she was taking 15 mg of Adderall, less than the prescribed 20, and her pain was much diminished. She reported more energy and restoration of sleep. Her dreams had diminished, and also, she was much less clumsy.

"Dr. Cochran, I have gone on the Internet to learn about narcolepsy, and I am sure I have cataplexy. I just didn't realize it when you asked me. I have had several times where my knees will just buckle for no reason causing me to grab hold of something to keep from falling."

"Well that is interesting. It is one more clue that you have narcolepsy although I don't think we really needed it. Your response to the Adderall, in my opinion, is virtually diagnostic."

"I have read your book, Dr. Cochran, and there was something in there that we didn't talk about. I have nocturia. Since I have become painful, I've had to get up six to eight times every night to empty my bladder. As soon as I started taking the Adderall, it cut down to just one or two times a night. I couldn't believe it. I thought I had bladder trouble. My bladder is working fine now."

"That's interesting, Lori, but I have to tell you it is not rare. I see many people who have nocturia with pain. I see it go away when pain is relieved. It can be quite a remarkable change."

Lori was under my care for only a few months before she and her family moved to another city. On her last visit, I joked with her a bit and told her she was the best-looking Sprengel's I had ever seen, but she was also the only Sprengel's I had ever seen. She liked that.

"Dr. Cochran, I can't tell you how much better I feel. I still have to take the Hydrocodone a couple of times a day although you told me I could take much more. I have no bad dreams at all, I have had no more cataplexy, and I am not clumsy anymore. I would not have believed this possible when I first came to see you."

"I am happy for you. One last question—how about the voidings at night?"

"Gone, totally gone, but I need to tell you something. I am taking three of the Adderall pills now. If I forget and miss one, just one mind you, I will have to get up through the night to empty my bladder."

Reader, I have written about connecting the dots, and with the knowledge of the bipolar spectrum, there are a lot more dots to connect. Just think about Lori. From a congenital deformity to depression to pain to narcoleptic dreams and cataplexy and for Pete's sake, nocturia! All are connected with each other. It is hard to understand, but it is real.

Carolyn was fifty-one, and she had suffered years of painful neuropathy. She was a registered nurse, and she carried an impressive résumé with high administrative posts at several area hospitals—administrative because her painful feet did not allow her to stand or walk for any length of time. She had been under the care of a pain clinic for some thirteen years and psychiatric care for depression for eight. She had undergone successful gastric bypass surgery with a hundred-pound weight loss. Unfortunately the weight loss did not diminish her pain when she stood or walked for any time. When she came to me she was taking extended release morphine 100 mg every eight hours.

"Carolyn, why are you coming to see me now after thirteen years at another pain clinic?"

"They discharged me."

"After thirteen years they terminated you? What was the reason?"

"My urine test was positive for drugs that they were not giving me—Hydrocodone and Oxycodone."

"Who was giving you those medicines?"

"My dentist gives me Hydrocodone and occasionally my primary care doctor, who knows me well and has been my doctor for many years, will give me a few Oxycodone to help with the breakthrough pain."

"Under the terms of your drug contract, the pain clinic had the right to fire you. Is that correct?"

"Yes, they had every right to do it, I suppose."

"But after thirteen years? How much of the drugs were you taking?"

"Really not many, maybe two or three pills a week."

"Why did the pain clinic not give you those drugs? Did you ask for them?"

"Well, I had asked them a few weeks ago to increase my Morphine, and they did. I went from 240 mg of morphine to 300 a day. They seemed reluctant to do that, and I was afraid to ask for any more opiate."

"So you went to other doctors?"

"Yes, that is what I did."

"Only two or three pills a week?"

"Yes."

"Are you angry?"

"Yes."

A word now about the urine drug screen. It would seem to be a convenient way to determine a patient's compliance. That is, whether they are taking the prescribed medicines appropriately. It is not nearly so simple. The different opiates have very similar chemical structures, and their metabolism is quite variable. Therefore, one opiate can be metabolized or converted to another one, and that will appear in the urine providing a high order of misinformation. Moreover, false positives are not infrequent. The common decongestant, Sudafed, for example, can appear in the urine as methamphetamine and a poppy seed roll as morphine. The American Pain Society, insurers, and regulating agencies mandate the necessity of obtaining urine drug screens to ensure patient compliance. I had given up on urine drug screens because I believe there are better ways to assure compliance, but now I am obliged to perform them routinely, and I often end up more confused coming out than I was going in.

Now let's again address the fear, suspicion, and misunderstanding that is such a barrier between the pain doctor and his patient. The doctor was distrustful of Carolyn's request for more opiates and supplied them only with hesitation. Carolyn, for her part, was distrustful of her doctor and fearful of telling him what she really needed because he would deem her a drug-seeker. It is this lack of open communication that is probably the greatest single barrier to the successful treatment of the person with chronic pain, and I have written that before.

I have been around long enough to know that Carolyn would carry this same distrust to me. She had been burned once, and she didn't want it to happen again, so she played her cards very close to the vest.

"Dr. Cochran, I am doing really rather well with the Morphine. I request that you prescribe that for me. I will be a very compliant patient and will request no other medicines from you. The Morphine will be just fine."

I knew she was lying, but it is not unusual for me to have patients come from other pain clinics advising to me that they are doing quite well on their current therapy, and that they need no change.

"Very well, Carolyn. I will write you the Morphine as you request, and I will make no changes in your therapy, but I would like to see you again in a month because I think we could be a little more imaginative."

On her return, she said to me, "Dr. Cochran, I have read your books, and I see a lot of myself in them. I am ready for you to push the envelope a little bit. Let me tell you some things about me that we didn't talk about on the first visit. We should have, but there is a lot about me that I didn't think you needed to know. I want to tell you I didn't have much of a childhood. There was no real abuse, mostly neglect. I was an A student and an achiever, and I have continued to achieve in spite of the neuropathy and the pain. The thing I most wanted to tell you is that I have nocturia. Six or seven times a night I get up to empty my bladder. Also, I have restless legs, night sweats, and a problem with grinding my teeth. I do it throughout the night and often bite myself and spit up blood in the morning. And, Dr. Cochran, I do have a real problem with breakthrough pain. The Morphine is simply not controlling it."

"Okay, Carolyn, we will give it a shot. We can't do everything at once though, but I am going to start you on some Imipramine and Klonopin. I want to see what that does for the pain and also the nocturia and all the rest. I will see you back in three weeks."

"I'll be here, and one other thing, Dr. Cochran. After I read your book, I really believe I have cataplexy. I am having more and more falls. I thought they were just due to my neuropathy, but I have researched it, and I do think I have cataplexy."

"Do you have vivid dreams?"

"Only when I was on Lexapro."

"Daytime sleepiness?"

"A little."

She was to tell me later that the effect had been dramatic. Her restless legs, night sweats, *bruxism* (teeth grinding), and nocturia had all suddenly abated. Some of this was comprehensible for we often use Imipramine to treat *enuresis* (bedwetting) in children. Maybe that was the accountant for part of her improvement. Why everything else should get so much better is very hard for me to understand. Nonetheless, I do accept that her symptoms were expressions of her disease, chronic pain, and perhaps, bipolarity.

"By the way, Carolyn, what has happened to your cataplexy?"

"It's gone. I haven't had a fall or stumble since I saw you."

"Do you need something more for pain?"

She turned her eyes down and said "Yes, I really do."

It took several weeks to find the right drug. A Fentanyl tablet, which dissolves in the mouth, gave her good benefit, but it was prohibitively expensive. We tried Oxycodone, which was ineffective and then, finally, immediate release morphine, which has given her very good pain control. She has told me some interesting things. She says that if she is on her feet a lot, she will have more pain, which is understandable. However, when she has more pain she will also have night sweats, which is much less so. She also tells me that if she goes without the Imipramine, the bruxism and restless legs come back. If she goes without the Klonopin, the night sweats and nocturia come back. The physician reader will recognize that all this is really quite unfathomable, but I see and hear the unfathomable almost every day. Chronic pain is a vast and complex disease, and I am astonished by the variety of its symptoms and astonished also by our ability, with appropriate therapy, to control so many of them.

Now back to Carolyn's discharge from the pain clinic. She was fired after thirteen years of compliance and appropriate urine drug screens. This strikes me as abrupt and, frankly, unwarranted. Thirteen years and a slip-up! And a minor one at that. Should we not temper justice with mercy? If there no place for compassion and trust? Well, nonetheless it had a happy ending. Her discharge from the pain clinic brought her to me and, it would seem, a cure.

Carolyn and I have been into her recovery about a year now. It has gone so well that she felt empowered enough to seek a very attractive position that was opening up in another hospital. Her credentials were impeccable, but she was told under no circumstances would she be considered for the post if she was taking opiates on a regular basis.

Trigeminal neuralgia is pain from the sensory nerve of the face and is one of the better defined states of pain, or at least it used to be. It is also known as *tic douloureux* (painful tic) referring to the facial grimaces that attend the lightning-like pain it engenders. It is characterized by intense, brief attacks of pain on one side of the face. It is often triggered by some facial movement such as chewing, and I remember well a patient from many years ago whose dour countenance was not a reflection of her emotional state but rather her knowledge that the act of smiling would unleash her tic douloureux.

The actual cause of trigeminal neuralgia is uncertain. It does appear with some frequency in people with multiple sclerosis. In some cases it is thought to be due to compression of the trigeminal nerve by a pulsatile artery. There is a surgical procedure known as *microvascular decompression* in which a cushion, often of Teflon, is placed between the artery and the nerve. It works some of the time.

Tic douloureux, by strict definition, is characterized by brief recurrent, lancinating pain in the face. But strict definitions are like the tip of the iceberg just as they are with bipolarity, ADD, OCD, and all the rest. Many people suffer from strange and usually undiagnosable face pains that are probably not true tics. Testament to this is the fact that the Trigeminal Neuralgia Association (TNA), a support group for those so afflicted, has changed its name to Trigeminal Neuralgia and Facial Pain Association (TNFPA).

Ralph was age fifty-four, gray, handsome, and extraordinarily articulate and personable. He began his career path studying for the ministry, but he ended up in the insurance business. Four years before coming to me he experienced the sudden onset of well localized pain in his right ear. He consulted an ENT specialist and was given a shot of cortisone. For a year he had no more pain. Then on the anniversary of his first pain, it reappeared. It was still predominant in the right ear but had spread to the upper face. Pain would wax and wane, and it lacked one of the defining attributes of classic tic in that it would last for several hours at a time. Nonetheless, a diagnosis of trigeminal neuralgia was made, and he was started on treatment with a variety of anticonvulsants, which were unhelpful. When he came to me he was taking Neurontin, Cymbalta, and the anti-inflammatory drug, Indocin. He had also recently been given an anesthetic eardrop, which controlled his pain quite well but only for a week or so. He had been offered surgical decompression, but he told me that he was not quite ready to have somebody enter his brain yet.

As is almost invariably the case, his past personal and social history were interesting and clue-giving. As a youngster he had been very active in school affairs. He enjoyed the academic work. Each summer when school was out, he would begin to feel depressed. He was three times married and divorced. His first and briefest was to a verbally abusive and probably very unstable woman because on more than a few occasions, she threatened him with bodily harm. Following the divorce, he told me he felt "hunted." He became quite fearful, especially at night. This lasted for some two years and then abated.

"How are you sleeping, Ralph?"

"Usually pretty well, but I do have to get up four or five times each night to empty my bladder."

"Does your pain ever strike in the middle of the night?"

"Yes, sometimes."

"Do you dream?"

"No."

"Are you depressed?"

"Yes, I am getting depressed. I am missing more time from work. This thing is really frustrating to me. You may be interested in something that is very queer to me. Every time I have an attack of pain, I have a sudden overwhelming depression. It will last for a few hours."

"How often does that happen?"

"Maybe two or three times a week."

"Do you ever get speeded up, have times where your mind works too fast?"

"Yes, sometimes I don't need sleep. I get very creative and energetic. I can work and get a lot accomplished. I feel very good during those times, and I don't miss the sleep at all."

"Do you get sleepy during the day?"

"Yes, it is very strange. Sometimes after a siege of pain, usually when it is going away, I become intensely sleepy."

"You say pain makes you sleepy?"

"Yes, and it happens quite a lot."

"How about your memory and mental focus?"

"It is really becoming a problem. I have trouble organizing my thoughts but, like I told you, there are times when I become very focused and creative."

"Are those episodes related to pain flares?"

"No, I don't think so."

Once again, bits and pieces of the bipolar spectrum. Mood shifts, ADD, and truly bizarre attacks of depression and sleep precipitated by ear pain. And to top it off, nocturia. Lots of dots. I prescribed Adderall.

It didn't take long at all. On his follow-up visit, he reported much diminution in his ear pain. He was no longer having sleep attacks. He felt less depressed, and his nocturia had diminished to two or three awakenings each night. Curiously, for a few days, as his ear pain diminished, he began to experience pain at the tip of his penis. It went away, he told me, after a week or so. Pain migrating from his ear to his penis—how in the world do we explain that? Only by accepting that the brain is a complex place that is constantly processing sensory input, and that it sometimes mislocates pain is understandable. This is the phenomenon of *referred pain*. The classic example is the man with coronary artery disease experiencing pain not in his chest but in his left arm or jaw or back. Even so, from the ear to the penis is quite a stretch, and I have not heard complaints like that very much at all.

Ralph has done nicely for several months now. With wellness, he has reordered his life and his priorities. He told me he did occasionally feel depressed, but that was because he was overwhelmed by the obligations and opportunities that health had afforded him. He had entered counseling, which he told me was quite helpful. He is essentially cured. No more nocturia, no more sleep attacks, better mental focus and attention, and thankfully, no more ear pain—none at all. He tells me he has returned to his studies for the ministry.

William was only twenty-nine when he came to me. He was married with children, and he worked in a manufacturing plant. He had two pain problems. One was migraine that had begun five years before. He told me he kept a dull headache over his left temple, and that two or three times a week it would become quite severe. It usually lasted twenty-four hours, but occasionally it would last two or three days. He had been prescribed Imitrex but had to discontinue the drug because it gave him chest pain. He also had low back pain radiating into both hips. On occasion his left leg would give out. He had no strength in it at all, and that would last for several minutes.

He had already been on multiple opiates including Hydrocodone, Oxycodone, and Morphine. They were helpful excepting those intervals where we would have sieges of back pain lasting up to ten days. When that happened, he developed enuresis and on occasion daytime urinary incontinence. With his sieges he would develop a disposition change—becoming very depressed and angry. He reported occasional intervals where his pain would diminish greatly. During these times he felt energized, and his mind was full of good ideas. He reported lifelong vivid dreams causing him to awaken frightened and emotional and sometimes briefly paralyzed. He also suffered sleep attacks during the day. His brother was an unstable bipolar. I prescribed Ritalin.

It was to be eighteen months before William achieved any semblance of recovery. It was a rollercoaster ride with a few highs and plenty of lows. Interestingly, with the Ritalin, he experienced near complete cessation of his migraines, but his back pain was, if anything, worse. I added Methadone. He reported that for a few days he felt quite well on the Methadone, but then he began to experience shortness of breath every time he took the pill, so he discarded it. On one of his visits he was actually in a pain siege, and I was able to witness its effects. He was sweaty, flushed, and obviously anxious and irritable. He had also entered a behavior change that I had not seen previously. He was catastrophizing, lamenting his fate and the certain knowledge that he would never get well. He was also, he told me, bedwetting again.

I tried Lithium, and that seemed to help some of his mood swings although not his pain, and it made his enuresis worse. Later, the mood-stabilizing antipsychotic Seroquel, which did nothing, and then a kindred drug, Abilify, which produced auditory hallucinations. No place to go but more opiate therapy. I increased the Oxycodone, and when we got up to the generous dose of 60 mg three times daily, he reported that his mood had stabilized, but his back pain diminished not at all. I suggested we try the Methadone again because, as we have certainly seen, it can be effective and well tolerated after initial failure. It produced shortness of breath, and his wife observed that on several occasions during his sleep he would stop breathing. He discontinued it and told me he didn't miss it at all. He did say, some six months into his treatment, that taking Oxycodone 60 mg every four hours let him feel more "positive" than in a long time, and with the combination of Ritalin and Oxycodone, his hypnagogic hallucinations had disappeared.

It was not to last. A few weeks later, a siege of back pain returned and with it enuresis and the appearance of vivid dreams. I gave him the opiate, Hydromorphone, one of our strongest. It did nothing. I increased his Oxycodone to 90 mg every four hours and wrote a prescription for Meperidine. I might as well keep trying, but I was becoming quite as frustrated as William. The Meperidine did nothing.

At this juncture I felt that sooner or later I was going to help William, probably by the administration of very high dosage opiates. I believe that there is a threshold that once achieved will cure, and I have written on this subject before. William had gotten up to 180 mg of Oxycodone every four hours—over a gram a day! He was better to be sure, but this was more with regard to mood than pain. He continued to have periodic sieges lasting days at a time during which he would again wet the bed and have bad dreams. And then a very good and very simple idea.

I have written many times in this book that *every* symptom must be recognized and, if possible, treated. You will recall that I have written that the bipolar spectrum gives us more points of attack, and that we should utilize any drug that might work. I had been treating William's bipolarity and pain with opiates. I had neglected to treat his enuresis. Could that possibly be a point of attack? I prescribed Imipramine, a drug that has been around over fifty years and that I employ almost invariably in those with chronic pain. I don't know why I had not used it sooner in William. I should have because it is a well-recognized treatment for enuresis in kids.

On his return, he looked much the best I had ever seen him. He was sleeping better at night and was no longer wetting the bed or suffering bad dreams.

"My pain is down to a five from an eight or nine, and I am doing more things around the house. My mood is good. I haven't had a migraine in months, and my legs are not giving out on me the way they used to."

"Do you think you can go back to work?"

"No, I am not near ready to go back to work. I still have too much pain."

"Okay, William, let's push the Imipramine dose on up and continue taking your Oxycodone and your Ritalin. Maybe we will get you out of this thing yet."

There was to be yet another dénouement and an improbable one at that.

"You look better, William. Are you feeling better?"

"Yes, I am feeling a lot better. I feel calmer, and my pain is better. It is down to a two or three now."

"That's wonderful. Frankly, William, it is astonishing to me that you would get this much benefit out of a drug like Imipramine. I should have started you on it a long time ago. I am sorry I didn't."

"Well, Doc, it is not just the Imipramine. You remember you had given me Methadone before. We tried it a couple of times, and although it helped me at first, it made me feel short of breath, so I stopped it. I found a bottle in the medicine cabinet and decided to try it one more time. It was wonderful. I feel better than I have in a long time."

"Any shortness of breath?"

"No, none at all."

The self-prescription of pharmacy. I can't condone it, but I accept the fact that my patients are going to experiment no matter what I tell them to do. As we have seen several times in this book, the results can be quite amazing.

William is a long way from well, but he is an even longer way from where we started. I anticipate that he will continue to improve, probably quite slowly, without any major change in his therapy. Some get better quickly, some slowly.

I am aware that many of the stories of those in pain that I write about may appear to be contrived. The suddenness and totality of recovery can often challenge credulity. William's recovery, or at least his approach to recovery, was neither sudden nor total, but it still challenges credulity that by attacking an issue peripheral to his pain, enuresis, with Imipramine, I was able to diminish his pain. And then the self-discovery that Methadone, a drug he had not tolerated before, was extremely helpful, almost curative.

There is a quality of *deus ex machina* about all this. For those of you unfamiliar with the term, it means, literally, "god out of a machine." It is a plot device first employed in the stage plays of the ancient Greeks. A seemingly inextricable problem is suddenly resolved with the introduction of a contrived agency in the form of magic or the hand of a god.

The stories I write are true. They are not contrived, but I will certainly not exclude the hand of God in their resolution.

CHAPTER 13

Craving

Edgar, at age fifty, came to me with chronic back pain. Like many bipolars, his life had been propelled by afterburners. He entered the military as a youngster and volunteered for Special Forces. Early on, during a training exercise, he witnessed the violent death of a close friend. The experience affected him deeply. He became depressed, anxious, and flashback-ridden. A military psychiatrist diagnosed post-traumatic stress disorder. Edgar eschewed psychiatric care and treated himself with alcohol and marijuana. His symptoms gradually abated as did his drug abuse.

After twenty years, during which time he had four marriages and three divorces, he concluded his military career. He completed his education and became a high school teacher and football coach. In his spare time he studied for the ministry and was appointed the pastor of a small church. These good things notwithstanding, his back pain progressively worsened as did his food cravings, and he became massively obese. His orthopedist felt that he needed a lumbar fusion but was fearful of the risk imposed by his obesity, diabetes, and hypertension. Edgar told his doctor that he was hopeful of getting gastric bypass surgery for weight loss. The orthopedist endorsed the operation and told Edgar that he would forgo any surgery on his back until his medical condition could be stabilized. He then referred him to me for pain management.

He was a truly massive man, some six feet in height and well over 350 pounds—the maximum my office scales can measure. He acknowledged he had always been a moody person and occasionally subject to suicidal ideation but never an attempt. He told me these feelings usually appeared when he was under stress and that also during those times he would feel quite irritable and angry. He acknowledged, in response to my questions, that he also experienced periodic hyperactivity and an inability to sleep. He told me that no doctor had ever said he was bipolar.

Note that some thirty years before, this man had treated his post-traumatic stress disorder by abusing drugs. Both of these are harbingers of the later development of chronic pain and perhaps bipolar disorder (my opinion). In earlier books, I wrote extensively about the role of drug abuse in the generation of chronic pain, and a brief review is appropriate. The scenario of drug abuse, recovery, and the subsequent development of chronic pain is quite common. The reasons for this are complex, and I will address this matter in the simplest manner possible. We must accept that alcohol can be pain-relieving, and there is no doubt about this observation. Alcohol stimulates the GABA neurotransmitter system, that which calms. However, the various neurotransmitter systems, and there are many of them, are highly interactive with one another, and enhanced GABA activity stimulates the opioid system. Thus, the analgesic property of alcohol is actually mediated by opioids. We know this because the administration of the opiate blocker, Naloxone, will diminish the analgesic effects of alcohol. (Naloxone is available in every emergency room in the country, and it is used to treat opiate overdosage.)

The alcoholic is constantly stimulating his opioid system artificially, and part of the good feeling that comes with alcohol is an opiate euphoria effect. When the alcoholic enters recovery, the brain's opioid system, accustomed to constant stimulation by alcohol, is deprived of that stimulus. After years of artificial stimulation, it has become insensitive to natural stimulation, and that is pain. Thus, the alcoholic in recovery is liable to experience chronic pain after injury or illness. All that said, we must acknowledge that Edgar's pain came on years removed from his alcohol abuse, and it is admittedly difficult to accept that after such a long time, his drug abuse was operative in the generation of his pain. Nonetheless, the appearance of chronic pain years removed from drug abuse occurs rather often.

I started his therapy conservatively, prescribing Imipramine and Klonopin. I maintained the Oxycodone prescribed by his orthopedist.

Edgar described good pain control and a certain sense of calmness with my therapy. He maintained his improvement and after numerous delays, he finally submitted to gastric bypass surgery. Prior the operation, he had the mandatory psychiatric consultation and was told that he was okay for surgery and that the drug therapy I had instituted two years before was quite satisfactory. He was also told that he had a "tendency to bipolarity."

The bypass operation was performed, and within the first month Edgar lost an astonishing seventy-two pounds. A problem, though. People who have bypass operations are often unable to take medications in tablet or capsule form. The medicine must be crushed or administered in liquid form in order to pass through the stomach into the digestive tract. Such was the case with Edgar. He crushed his Oxycodone and mixed it with applesauce. So far so good, and all was going well with Edgar. Then after a few months he presented me with another problem.

"I am craving the Oxycodone. It is not lasting long enough. I am having to take more of it."

"Tell me exactly what is happening. What do you feel when you take the Oxycodone?"

"I feel good. I have no pain, but that only lasts two or three hours and then I start getting nausea and sweats. They go away in just a few minutes if I take another Oxycodone pill. Am I becoming an addict?"

I cannot totally exclude the fact that his symptoms were due to rapid absorption of his drug by virtue of his altered gastrointestinal anatomy. More probably he was experiencing a true addiction. He was, in his own words, craving the Oxycodone. Its duration of effectiveness was diminished, and he had to have more to control his pain. The nausea and sweats were perhaps symptoms of opiate withdrawal.

Should I have sent him to an addictionologist, one expert in removing a person from opiates? That certainly would have solved my problem. I am not at all sure what it would have done for Edgar's. Remember, I was treating not only his pain but also his bipolarity with the Oxycodone. I chose to add Methadone, the craving-relieving opiate.

It worked quite well, indeed, astonishingly well. His pain and his withdrawal symptoms abated totally, and he no longer experienced cravings for his Oxycodone. Recall that I have already written about several people in whom the addition of Methadone to prior opiate therapy relieved pain and diminished cravings.

A digression here to develop an idea. Edgar's cravings might have represented an addiction, but there are other explanations. Perhaps he was developing *tolerance* to his Oxycodone. This phenomenon is quite common with opiates, thus the reason for the escalation of dosage to achieve the same effect. Tolerance usually develops slowly, but in Edgar's case it appeared over the course of but a very few weeks. Another explanation is that he had developed *opioid-induced hyperalgesia.* In this state, the opiate gives relief of pain for a few hours followed by the appearance of an even worse pain, the *hyperalgesia* (more pain). This effect appears to be mediated through opiate stimulation of a certain glutamate receptor that I will identify, mercifully, in its acronymic form, NMDA.

Edgar got well with the Methadone because, remarkably, that drug was appropriate for any of the three conditions that I have listed. If his cravings represented an addiction, they could be controlled with Methadone, widely used for that purpose. If the cravings were due to increasing tolerance of the drug, the introduction of more opiate, in his case in the form of Methadone, or for that matter even more Oxycodone, would diminish the problem of tolerance by making more drugs available. And if his problem was indeed opiate induced hyperalgesia, Methadone would work because it will block NMDA receptors. The glutamate/NMDA axis is an excitatory mechanism that is probably responsible not only for opiate induced hyperalgesia but also such excitatory phenomena as panic, mania, migraine, and perhaps even flashbacks. Methadone is unique among the opiates in that it has a blocking effect on NMDA receptors. Almost no other opiate shares that property, and that is almost certainly the reason Methadone can be so useful for so many bad things. So, to conclude, it is increasingly difficult for me, and I suspect others, to identify just what addiction is and just who is addicted. The line between opiate tolerance, opiate induced pain, and opiate addiction is a vague one indeed.

Edgar did well for a matter of six months or so. During that interval he lost 130 pounds. He continued his active and productive lifestyle and returned to the seminary to obtain a master's degree. Such is bipolar velocity! Then a new and unforeseen problem.

"Dr. Cochran, something has happened to me. My disposition is changing. I feel irritable and angry all the time. I have had lots of arguments with people I shouldn't be arguing with. My congregation says I preach angry, and they tell me that I change like the weather. They are about ready to vote me out. I am getting real depressed, Doc. What can we do?"

"Edgar, you may remember that when you saw the psychiatrist before your bypass operation, he told you that you had a tendency to bipolarity. You do remember that, don't you?"

"Yes."

"Well, what you are having now is more than a tendency. This is your bipolar disorder coming to the surface. Your anger and your irritability are symptoms of that disease, and I think we may be able to control it by increasing both the Oxycodone and Methadone. If that doesn't work pretty well, I will have to send you to a psychiatrist."

"I will do what you say, Doc, but one more thing. I am having real bad dreams now. They are terrible. A lot of them are about my buddy who was killed when we were in the service together."

"Take the pills, Edgar, and hang on for the ride. I am hopeful we can get you better."

It worked for a while, a couple of months or so, and then Edgar's shifting moods took over again. I referred him to a psychiatrist.

The diagnosis of bipolar disorder was confirmed, and he was begun on treatment with Cymbalta and Seroquel. Relief from mood shifts, irritability, anger, and nightmares came rather quickly and, somewhat to my surprise, Edgar told me his psychiatrist had no problem at all with my therapy with Klonopin, Imipramine, Oxycodone, and Methadone. Polypharmacy to be sure, but sometimes that is what it takes.

Drew came to me on referral from his brother, a patient I had successfully treated for bipolarity and pain. He was an automobile salesman and an alcoholic. Some eight years before, after a DUI, he entered a treatment center. He stayed sober for six months and then relapsed. He was drinking at least ten beers daily, and he told me that beverage helped control his pain—and he had lots of it. He was facing replacements of both hips and following that a lumbar fusion for his progressive back pain.

"I know I am going to have a lot of pain through those operations, and I am having a lot of pain now. You helped my brother a lot. Can you help me?"

"Yes, I can probably help you, but you are going to have to help me. I can give you opiates for pain relief, but if you mix them with alcohol you can get in trouble—big trouble."

"I will work with you, Doc, but we have to talk about some things. I know I am bipolar. I am just like my brother. He has it, and I am sure I have it."

"Tell me about it."

"Well, I have been depressed all my life, and I think that may be why I drink. My moods are all over the place. There are times when I feel good, and then the least thing will upset me and I will slip into a deep depression. I am fearful and anxious a lot, and sometimes I spend money foolishly, for no real reason at all. And I have attacks of anger and rage. It doesn't happen a lot, but when it does, it is not pretty. That sounds like bipolar disease, doesn't it?"

"Yes, it does. How are you sleeping at night?"

"I can't."

"Why?"

"I can't turn my mind off. I have racing thoughts that keep me from going to sleep. I also have bad dreams. They really are horrible. I have had them all my life, and they scare me. They seem so real."

"Do you get sleepy during the day?"

"Yes, and that is becoming more of a problem. And I am fatigued. I am really tired all the time."

"Drew, I am going to try to help you, but I must emphasize again that there is great risk when you mix opiates with alcohol. I am going to give you some Oxycodone for pain and some Klonopin to help your sleep and maybe arrest those dreams. I am hopeful they can control your mood also, but you are the one who is going to have to control the drinking. Maybe if we can control your pain and your bipolarity, you will have less craving for alcohol. I hope it plays out that way, but I am by no means certain. So a lot of this is going to be up to you."

When he returned he told me he was sleeping better, and that his hip and back pain were much relieved. However, he was continuing to have trouble with depression, mood shifts, and fatigue. He told me also that he had cut down on his drinking quite a lot. I wrote him a prescription for Adderall in addition to the Oxycodone and Klonopin.

When I saw him next he had undergone the first hip replacement and was, with my medicines, doing quite well. He told me his thinking was better, and his energy was much improved. He said the Adderall "evens me out." He also told me "I am living a different life. I am not angry anymore."

Drew returned early for his next appointment. The reason, he said, was that he had an appointment to see his orthopedist that day, and since he lived some distance away, it would be convenient to see me also. He told me that he was "100 percent better," that he was drinking a lot less beer, and that he was taking my medicines exactly as scheduled. He was lying to me as I was to discover on his next visit, also premature.

"I am sorry, Doc, but I am out of medicine. I am using more of it, and I have to tell you that I am craving it. To be honest with you, Doc, it is the same craving I have for alcohol. I just have to have it. I can't get by without it."

"Which drug are you craving, Drew? The Oxycodone or the Adderall?"

"Both of them."

I added Methadone.

He was smiling broadly, and he looked vastly better than I had ever seen him before. His pain was well controlled, he told me, and he felt an emotional calmness that he had never known before.

"Drew, how about the Oxycodone and Adderall? Are you taking them as I prescribed?"

"Yes, absolutely. This is amazing, but I have no craving for them at all. I am taking them just as you told me."

"I hope you are telling me the truth, Drew."

"I am, Doc. I promise you I am."

And he probably was. The change that comes to these people is evident in their appearance and their behavior. It's "the sky is blue again" effect. Such recovery cannot be feigned. It is irrefutable evidence, and even the most casual observer can't miss it.

"Doc, there is something else I have got to tell you."

"What's that?"

"I have stopped drinking. I have no craving for alcohol at all. Did the Methadone do that?"

"Well, Drew, I have never heard it before, but I can see how it could happen."

"Can I stay on these medicines, Doc?"

"Yes."

Methadone arrested cravings for Oxycodone. That effect is well known. However, the arrest of cravings for the stimulant, Adderall, and alcohol was new to my experience. I had never heard of it, but I have since learned from a counselor at a methadone maintenance clinic that several of her clients told her that Methadone arrested their cravings for alcohol. So I suppose the effect is real.

I saw Drew next in the company of his wife and brother. He was obviously troubled, tremulous and anxious. His wife had a look of steely anger and his brother one of resignation. I knew right away that Drew had been overusing his medicine and was in a withdrawal. I initiated conversation and, as usual in these events, each party told me a somewhat different story. Piecing it all together as best I could, it seemed that Drew had been doing well with the Methadone, craving neither alcohol, Adderall, nor Oxycodone. But then he began to experience one of the side effects of ongoing Methadone therapy, and that is sedation. He even fell asleep during the family's Christmas dinner with his face falling into his plate. At his wife's insistence, he discontinued his Methadone, and within a few days his cravings for alcohol, Oxycodone, and Adderall all returned.

I told Drew that a referral to an addictionologist or a treatment center was mandatory. In a brief moment of agreement, both Drew and his wife said he couldn't do it right now. He had important business matters to attend to and also a troubled son in jail after repeated DUIs. I gave him a prescription for a month's supply of the Oxycodone and Adderall and told his wife that she must administer the drugs to Drew. I advised them that I was terminating his care. They would have to see the addictionologist within the timeline of one month. If they were unable to do so, he would go into withdrawal for which I would provide no more medicine. Drew and his wife left the room, in demeanor and body language expressing their intense anger for each other. His brother, who has been my patient for many years and whom I consider my friend, stayed behind and whispered to me, "This will be his third detox."

"I doubt that it is going to work."

"You are right. It is not."

Drew was, by any standard of measure, an addict. He could not control his cravings for alcohol, for Oxycodone, or for Adderall. I wish I could have done a better job with him. I do believe that it is likely that the Methadone could have controlled his cravings had he been able to tolerate it. There may be another point of attack. It is just possible that Drew's bipolar disorder, and remember, this had never been diagnosed before he came to me, could be controlled with pharmacy. It just might control his addiction because I do believe there is a link between addiction and bipolarity.

Some more thoughts on the complex issue of drug abuse and addiction in those taking opiates for pain. First of all, be advised that there is general agreement among authorities in pain management that a past history of drug abuse does not preclude the use of painkilling opiates if medically necessary. That is to say, a person in pain should not be deprived of pain relief simply on the basis of past indiscretions. One would think that the re-emergence of addictive behavior would be quite common. In my experience, this is not the case at all. It certainly was in Drew but he is, I believe, an exception. To put this in some sort of perspective, the need for intervention, that is, detoxification and aftercare by a trained professional occurs in my practice rather infrequently. Maybe six or eight times a year a patient will come to me, almost always in the company of family, because of blatant drug abuse and addiction and with it the need for referral to an addictionologist. Other patients of mine end up with interventions by virtue of overdosing on their drugs and requiring a hospital admission where their drug abuse is recognized and treated. There is yet another group of patients, those that I have discharged from my care because of undisciplined and erratic filling of their opiate prescriptions. I do not know, since I have no follow-up, how many of these patients are truly addicted and how many are selling their drugs for profit. I would estimate that perhaps twenty to thirty of my patients require discharge from my care each year. This may seem like quite a lot, but be aware that my patient population totals nearly two thousand souls. Thus, the annual incidence of addictive behavior in my patients amounts to one to 1.5 percent, which is pretty much in the middle of the nationally reported 0.5 to 3 percent incidence of addiction in those taking opiates for pain. The risk is there to be sure, but it is not nearly as bad as you might think.

Be advised that some of my patients who are dependent upon opiates for relief of pain but who are by no means addicted do occasionally request withdrawal from the drugs. These requests are almost always at the behest of family members who consider opiate therapy as stigmatizing and shameful. Thus, opiates are a convenient culprit for any of the emotional and behavioral hiccups that we human beings all experience. Any deviation from customary behaviors in a person taking opiates is, in the minds of many, prima-facie evidence that the victim is opiate-addicted, and I will return to that subject soon. I must remind you also that many interventions are the product of threatening circumstances, and I am referring to job loss, divorce, and child custody. Lastly, let me advise you that taking more pills than prescribed is not necessarily addiction. I have already given many examples throughout this book, and I will again in the next case study.

"Bob, I am referring my patient Larry Swift to you for pain management. He broke his wrist playing ball about eighteen months ago. He really had a bad injury. I operated on him and had to put in some hardware to stabilize the fracture. He didn't do well, and I had to re-operate. He kept having pain, and I did a third operation, fusing the joint, just a few months ago. He is still hurting and asking for more Oxycodone than I am willing to prescribe. He sure doesn't need another operation. I would like to turn him over to you. Can you see him for me?"

"Sure."

Larry had a very flat affect, and his limited speech was slow and monotonous, devoid of emotional content. His wife entered the conversation early on. She was concerned over his use of the Oxycodone. He had to take more than prescribed, and she was fearful that he was becoming an addict.

"Are you craving the drug, Larry?"

"I don't think I am craving the medicine. I am craving the relief. I can function when I have the medicine. If I don't, I can't function at all. I hurt too much."

"Larry, we have got to let the doctor know you have been getting pain medicine from several of your friends."

"Okay, I'll admit I have done that."

I reviewed his medical history and learned that he had been on Celexa for six years. This was begun after what he called an "anxiety breakdown." He had, at age thirty-five, suddenly developed intense anxiety. He became sleepless at night, subject to mind-racing. He was so incapacitated that for two weeks he could barely get out of bed. His physician prescribed Celexa, and within but a few days his anxiety went away, and he was able to return to his work as a civil engineer.

Let's pause briefly now and note that at the age of forty he suffered an injury to his wrist, and a serious one at that. He had been surgically stabilized, and he should have recovered, but he did not. Failure to recover from injury and the subsequent development of chronic pain is, I believe, a clue to bipolarity. Was his "anxiety breakdown" years before an episode of bipolar mania? It surely could have been. I pursued my inquiries.

"Larry, are your moods up and down?"

"No, not at all. I am very even."

Injected his wife, "He is even to the point of torpor. He doesn't get up, and he doesn't get down at all."

"Are you depressed, Larry?"

"No I am not depressed, but I have to admit I have never been happy, and I really don't like being around people most of the time. Coming to see you is making me kind of nervous."

"Has anxiety been a problem for you along the way?"

"Most of the time, no, since starting the Celexa, but I do have what I am told is anticipatory anxiety. Even as a kid, when I was assigned a certain task, I would become nervous to the point of nausea. Once I started on the task, it would suddenly go away. I play golf with my father and before we start, I always get anxious and sometimes have to vomit. Once I start playing, it all goes away, and I enjoy myself."

"Okay, let's get to the Oxycodone now. How much are you taking?"

"I take six of the 10 mg pills a day."

"Is that what Dr. Hogan prescribed?"

"No, he prescribed just four a day, but I have to have more."

"Does the Oxycodone relieve your pain?"

"Only for two or three hours."

"Does it do anything else for you? Does it affect you in any other way—either for the good or the bad?"

His wife again. "He really becomes more social and more conversational after he takes the Oxycodone. I have noticed it, and I worry about that. Is it a sign of addiction? I am afraid the medicine is working too well."

Did my patient need to come off his drug because it made him feel better, or because it made him feel better did he need more of it? I much favor the latter. I told Larry and his wife that I was going to increase the dose of his Oxycodone beyond the six pills a day he was taking. I was doing that to relieve his pain and, if in the process of doing that I could make him more social and conversational, there is nothing wrong with that.

Larry and his wife returned at the appointed time. He appeared as flat and as emotionally impoverished as he did on the first visit, and I surprised when he told me with no enthusiasm at all that he was 80 percent better. His pain was much diminished, and he wasn't as "unhappy as I used to be." Well, progress of a sort. I surmised that Larry had never been an enthusiastic person and probably, even with therapy, never would be. His wife, however, told me that she could see a big improvement in his energy and demeanor. They were actually talking with each other more, and she was quite happy about that.

I had partially controlled his pain with Oxycodone. Could I make him even less painful and less unhappy with a bigger dosage? I wrote a prescription.

Larry was in a bad way when he returned. The date was May 12, 2010. It was a momentous time for my city and for Larry. His downtown office where he kept half of his Oxycodone pills was underwater after the flood hit on May 1. This was understandably an anxiety-producing event that Larry didn't handle very well. He should have called me. I was not underwater, and I could have written him another prescription as I did for many of my patients who were flood-damaged. But Larry, for whatever reason, decided to tough it out. It didn't work. With a limited supply of Oxycodone on hand, he became increasingly anxious. He discovered that taking more of the Oxycodone would calm him. He exhausted his supply and then went into opiate withdrawal. He required a visit to an emergency room where a thoughtful physician wrote him a prescription for Oxycodone and instructed him to get to me right away.

"Dr. Cochran, I was doing real good on the bigger dose of Oxycodone. I mean really good. But after the flood I began craving the drug. I just had to have more and more of it. And then the opiate withdrawal—that was just horrible."

"You should have called me, Larry, you really should have. I was available, and I would have given you more medicine."

"I know, but I didn't want to call you. I was afraid you would be upset that I was taking more of the medicine."

"Well, I might have been, but that is unimportant now. I want us to start over. I am going to write you a prescription for the Oxycodone at an even bigger dose, 60 mg four times daily. Take it exactly as instructed, and I am hopeful that you are going to do well."

Larry returned before his scheduled appointment. He was more animated than I had seen him before. He told me that for the first couple of weeks on the Oxycodone he felt just great. He was free of pain, he was not unhappy at all, and he was functioning quite well at work. Then he started becoming anxious and fearful of running out of his Oxycodone. He would awaken at night with anxiety and take another pill. He was, he admitted, obsessing and fearful about running out of his medicine.

"Larry, are you craving the Oxycodone?"

"I don't think I am craving Oxycodone, I think I am craving relief."

"Well, Larry, I don't see how you can be an addict two weeks out of a month and not the other two weeks. I have to tell you your fears of running out of the medicine are groundless. I will be here for you, and if I am not here there will be somebody else. I can promise you that I will provide the medicines if you take them as I instruct."

He returned in three weeks, not the appointed four. His high anxiety was quite evident.

"It happened again. The first two weeks were just fine, and then I started worrying about running out of medicine. The only way to stop the worry was to take more. Can you give me another prescription and write on it that it can be filled early? Otherwise, my pharmacy won't fill it."

"Larry, I will do that for you, but I am not going to keep doing this. I am going to add some Methadone. It can sometimes relieve cravings for other opiates, and it looks to me like that is what is happening to you. I don't know why it should happen just two weeks out of four, but this is the next step to take. If this doesn't work, I have got to get you to an addictionologist, and I will no longer participate in your care."

He kept his four-week appointment. He looked quite well—the best I had seen him. The Methadone, I surmised, had done it again.

"You look well, Larry."

"I am well, Dr. Cochran. I am really doing good."

"You took the Oxycodone exactly like I told you?"

"Yes, exactly."

"And the Methadone?"

He handed me his prescription bottle full of Methadone pills and for the first time actually smiled at me. He told me he had not taken the first one.

"I have got it figured out. I really have it figured out now. I really wasn't craving the Oxycodone. What was happening to me was anticipatory anxiety. It was the same thing I experienced when I played softball or golf, although it was much worse. As soon as I got to thinking about coming back to see you, I would get very nervous and fearful. You may not like this, Dr. Cochran, but you are my stressor. It is fear of not having you and not having the Oxycodone that was giving me anxiety. When I realized this, I told myself I could control that feeling and that fear, and I was able to."

Amazing. That which looked like addiction with cravings and drug abuse was in reality only anticipatory anxiety. Larry figured it out himself. He did it without my assistance, and that is good.

Larry continues to do well. He tells me that he is more social and conversational and also more carefree and spontaneous. On a recent weekend, he decided, on impulse, to take his family to an air show. It was a delightful experience for all, and he was looking forward to more such occasions when he did things spontaneously because he was less unhappy.

I wanted to make sure to include Larry's story in this book as much for me as for you. In my enthusiasm for pharmacy and the miracles that can be achieved with it, I sometimes forget that human intelligence and will can be powerful weapons against illness. I helped Larry's pain and his bipolar disorder with Oxycodone. He was the one who cured his anticipatory anxiety and his opiate craving.

I want to share with you a couple of paragraphs from a long letter that Larry sent me describing his unhappy life.

Baseball was the most important thing in the world to me. I loved to watch the pros, and I must admit, I imitated them as I played youth baseball. To my knowledge, my bouts with anxiety started with baseball. Prior to each game

I became nauseous. I could not eat before games. I did not even want to talk with anyone. My arms would tremble, my legs were weak, and the smell of a concession stand hotdog made me puke more than once. However, when the game started all symptoms vanished. That is when all was right with the world. Once the first pitch was thrown, I would be all right. So it was not the game that stressed me out, it was the anticipation. It was the waiting. It was the thinking. I call it Anticipatory Anxiety.

Now I don't know if anticipatory anxiety is a medically recognized disorder. However, for me, it has been a fact of life since little leagues. Just the mere thought of preparing for event that would happen in the near future, even a good one, made me a nervous wreck. Prior to golf matches, the drive to the golf course was excruciating. I trembled, was nauseated, and had terrible bouts of diarrhea. If I had to be somewhere at a designated time, like getting to a restaurant to meet someone or having to be somewhere for a meeting, the same symptoms would crop up. It started immediately with diarrhea then turned into nausea to the point that the smell of food would make me sick. Finally, there was the uncontrollable shaking of my arms and legs and weakness in my knees. It was debilitating. Strangely enough though, once I made the first tee shot at the golf course or finally made it to my destination, all the symptoms of anxiety diminished. I mean completely vanished. Anticipatory anxiety has controlled my entire life.

A segment of another letter, this from a young bipolar whose life was restored with Methadone but who, by virtue of his encounters with me, also suffered anticipatory anxiety.

I spoke with you about my fears of running out of medicine early or that the pharmacy might be closed, just an endless number of imaginary sensations that seemingly could happen. After speaking with you, however, and realizing that it was not just me but that others had the same problem, I tried just accepting that everything was going to be fine, and it absolutely worked out fine—just as you said it would.

I think that in the course of my treating and often curing those in pain, I have created a small epidemic of anticipatory anxiety. Larry told me that I was his stressor. Priscilla, in the chapter "Cutting and Biting," used the very same words. She became anxious to the point of mutilating herself for relief before she came to see me for fear that I would not be available for her. When I relieve the pain, I also create the fear that recovery will be lost if I am not available. The anxiety it induces, as we have seen, can be severe. It is really not uncommon at all. It can be a very disabling condition and certainly an unforeseen outcome of recovery.

Before concluding this chapter, I want to introduce you to a very strange craving that I see not infrequently in those in pain. Please recall the story of Roger from the chapter "Dreams." He had back pain and was narcoleptic, and he craved cabbage, heavily salted. His lust for that food appeared when his back pain began and abated when I treated his pain, narcolepsy, and attention deficit disorder with Ritalin, Klonopin, and Hydrocodone. At the time of this writing Roger is doing well, and he tells me that although he continues to enjoy heavily salted cabbage, he doesn't eat it more than a serving a week, which is nothing compared to the two heads that he consumed every week when he was in pain.

April was sixty-one, working part-time in retail sales. She was three times married, currently for many years quite happily. She developed back pain following an automobile accident three years before and also fibromyalgia. She complained of chronic fatigue and sleeplessness and acknowledged some depression but said, "I live with it." She had been on Prozac for ten years, beginning the drug at the time she was the caregiver for her mother, ill with Alzheimer's. She described herself as a very restless person, and she had never been unable to sustain a desk job because she couldn't sit still for any length of time. She acknowledged also mind busyness and thought-racing and was increasingly frustrated because of trouble with mental focus and memory. She also reported that since she had become painful she was experiencing nocturia, awakening three times at night to void and, curiously, cravings for sweets and salt.

"Tell me about those cravings. Do you have them all the time, or do they come and go?"

"Oh, they come and go. They will strike me very suddenly, and sometimes it is sweets and sometimes it is salt."

"Do you crave chocolate?"

"Not especially, just anything sweet."

"Do you have cravings for sweets and salt at the same time?"

"No, it is one or the other."

"What happens when you satisfy your cravings? Does it change your mood or does it help your pain?"

"I'm not sure. I just know I feel a lot better when I satisfy a craving."

Sweet cravings are common in those in pain, thus the frequent problem with weight gain. One would think that chocolates would stand on a high order of cravings because they contain tyramine, the precursor of the mood-elevating neurotransmitter, serotonin. Curiously, however, very few of my pain-suffering patients have a specific craving for chocolates. More often it is carbohydrates and particularly sweets. And cravings for salt are not rare at all.

I prescribed Imipramine and Klonopin and, at her request, wrote a prescription for Darvocet. She had taken it in the past, she told me, and it had helped her.

She returned in but a few days to tell me that the Imipramine and Klonopin were diminishing her nocturia and also helping her sleep. The Darvocet, however, was ineffective in controlling pain. She then volunteered that she had misspoken (or perhaps I had misheard) and that the drug she wanted was Percocet. I prescribed it four times a day.

"That Percocet is marvelous. I am wearing shoes I haven't worn in two years because I haven't been able to bend over and tie them. My depression is much improved. And this is most curious, I don't have to get up to empty my bladder at all at night, and I have had absolutely no cravings for sweets or salts. Can you explain that to me?"

"No, I can't, but I suspect it may be important. You will be interested to know that you are not alone. I have several patients whose food cravings go away when their pain is relieved."

April and I have been at it for two years now. I have added Adderall for her attention deficit disorder, and she is doing extremely well with no recurrence of her nocturia or her sweet or salt cravings.

I don't know what the appearance of sweet or salt cravings in those in pain and the disappearance of these cravings when cure is achieved really means, and I can only speculate, and that at the most primitive level. Perhaps the sweet cravings represent the body's search for energy, which is almost invariably lacking in those in pain. Unfortunately, the ingested sweets can't give energy. Instead, they are metabolically transformed into fat. Be aware that sodium and chloride, the components of table salt, are necessary, among other things, for the transmission of the electrical message through the length of the nerve cell, and perhaps the salt-craver is seeking better nerve cell performance to fight the pain. Sorry, that is the best I can do.

Donna was forty-three years old and self-employed as a hairdresser. She lost one of her sons in an automobile accident some three years before. Following that, she experienced worsening of her chronic low back pain and anxiety, and the appearance of vivid dreams, mostly related to her son's death. She was treated with Ativan, which she found extraordinarily helpful in relieving her anxiety and diminishing her dreams. She remained on it for several months until her doctors told her that she would have to quit taking it or else she would become an addict. Her anxiety, pain, and nightmares returned, and with them a craving for sea salt.

"Does it have to be sea salt? Do you crave table salt?"

"No, it just has to be sea salt. It is only thing that satisfies me. I feel calmer with sea salt."

"Can you describe it in any more detail than that?"

"No, I really can't. It is just a craving that I have. When the craving is fulfilled, I feel serene."

"Does sea salt do anything for your pain or your dreams?"

"No, but it does help my anxiety, and I have to have it. I can't explain it any better than that."

I prescribed Ativan for her and why not? It had helped her a lot, and I saw no need to deprive her of a drug that had been so beneficial. Again, her doctors were measuring proven benefit against the potential for harm. I come down strongly on the former. Why not use a drug that works, a drug that cures? I also gave her Hydrocodone for pain.

"Dr. Cochran, the Ativan has really been helpful. I am only taking it a couple of times a day. I know you wrote it for more than that, but I don't need it. I am sleeping better, and I am not nearly as anxious. I have to tell you, though, that the Hydrocodone just isn't working. I am taking it like you told me, six times a day, but I am just not getting much pain relief from it."

"I am going to change you to a stronger opiate, Donna. It is known as Oxycodone, and you can take it up to four times a day. By the way, let me ask you, have your salt cravings changed in any way?"

"No, not at all. I am still craving."

When she returned she told me that she responded quite well to the Oxycodone. Her pain was much diminished, and she said she had more things to tell me.

"Dr. Cochran, I have read your books, and there are some things I didn't tell you that I perhaps should have. I have had mood shifts all my life and was diagnosed with attention deficit disorder when I was a teenager. My mother wouldn't let me take Ritalin, though. Also, my son, the one who was killed, had attention deficit disorder, and he was on treatment with Adderall. One last thing, my mother is sure that I am bipolar. I just wanted to share that with you."

"Well, Donna, it all fits, and I am glad you told me. By the way, I am still interested in your salt cravings. Has anything happened?"

"Yes, a lot. I still like sea salt and I use it, but there is a difference, a definite difference. I don't crave it now, and I was craving it then. I like the taste of the sea salt, but it doesn't do anything for my emotions anymore. For a while there it made me feel serene."

Serene is a pretty strong word. I found no reason, no reason at all, to disbelieve what my patient was telling me. Sea salt cravings in those in pain are not uncommon (in those not in pain, I don't know). Again, let's speculate. Sea salt is an unrefined product. It contains salts not only of sodium but also other minerals such as potassium, magnesium, and, get this, lithium—the very drug we use to treat bipolar disorder. The quantity of lithium in sea salt is miniscule, far below the dosage we usually employ in the treatment of bipolar disorder. Still, one wonders.

A bipolar patient of mine regularly takes a proprietary preparation of mixed salts in solution. It contains, among other salts, lithium carbonate. She says she finds it very mood stabilizing. I calculate that the dose of lithium she is receiving is 10 mg a day. The usual start-up dose is 300 mg! I would never anticipate mood stabilization with the amount she was taking, but I cannot disbelieve her.

CHAPTER 14

Blaming

Anita came to me at age forty in 2005. She had been many months fibromyalgia painful and was taking Neurontin prescribed by her primary care doctor. She found that drug too sedating to take during the day, but it was very effective in improving her disordered sleep. She acknowledged depression at the time of her divorce ten years before. She was treated with Prozac. She denied depression currently but acknowledged that she was extremely frustrated and worried about her health. She also told me that she had suffered several years of anorexia as a teenager. I prescribed Nortriptyline, Klonopin, and Hydrocodone and maintained her Neurontin therapy.

On her first return visit, she was more candid with me. She told me she had read my books and was very excited about the ideas that I offered. She told me she had been in pain for many years with temporomandibular (jaw) joint disease and endometriosis. She also admitted a brutal rape at age seventeen and a physically and sexually abusive first marriage. She required treatment for several years for her post-traumatic stress disorder. She also volunteered that her thirteen-year-old daughter had attention deficiency. My medicine was helping her, she said. She was sleeping much better and was less anxious. This notwithstanding, she found herself frequently tearful and emotionally labile with mood shifts. She then offered the observation that for years she had been unable to cry. Now under the sponsorship of my therapy, she was doing it quite frequently.

The ability to cry in one who has been previously unable to is probably a pretty good sign. I viewed it as a return to, dare I use the word, a more normal emotionality. I added Cymbalta.

"The Cymbalta has helped a lot. I am more myself now. I am physically doing more, and I am not as depressed. I didn't realize just how depressed I was until I got on the Cymbalta."

"So it is going well, Anita?"

"Yes, very well indeed."

A year and half into treatment a major setback. Her daughter attempted suicide and was admitted to a psychiatric facility. She was diagnosed with bipolar disorder, and the family was in counseling.

Along the way, I obtained a urine drug screen test. It was appropriate for the drugs she was taking but also for marijuana. She told me she used it to relieve her pain, and that it was very effective.

"Dr. Cochran, I am definitely better than when we started, but still it seems that I worry a lot—about everything. My pain is tolerable 60 or 70 percent of the time, but I am getting more depressed."

At that juncture I elected to add Adderall. She found it very helpful. She had better mental focus and energy and felt less depressed.

My next encounter was a phone call from her husband telling me that they were at the emergency room, and that Anita was to be admitted because she was delusional and suicidal. I heard nothing more from her or her husband, or for that matter the hospital.

When I saw her next, some two months later, she told me that after an evaluation at the hospital she was discharged with no change in her medications. The whole thing, she said, was a family matter. She was exhausted and upset with her family, particularly her daughter. There was another issue, and a major one at that. With the Adderall she had no appetite at all. She was losing weight rapidly, and with her history of anorexia, she was fearful of remaining on the drug although it had been very helpful to her.

I discontinued the Adderall and prescribed Ritalin in its place, hopeful that she would get the same benefit without the appetite-suppressing effect. It worked pretty well, but she continued to be in pain and mood-shifty. She was better than when we started, but by no means had I achieved a cure. Why not try Methadone? I did, and it produced nausea and sedation. She was quite unable to tolerate it.

"Dr. Cochran, I have got a new complaint. It has been with me ever since I went to the hospital for that evaluation. I have a sense of numbness and electricity throughout my body. I have had symptoms like that before I came to see you, and for a while the doctors thought I had multiple sclerosis. They couldn't prove it though, and the symptoms went away until now. When I walk, my body feels like a tuning fork."

"It is painful?"

"No, it is not painful, but it is frightening and debilitating to me. I am feeling depressed again, and I have no energy, and I am not sleeping well."

What was going on with Anita? Clearly, she had a mood disorder, recurrent, and in the endgame, treatment resistant. She also had treatment-resistant pain. Now the development of a delusion, the belief in something that is not there. Or perhaps better, a sensory hallucination of feeling something that is not there. Anita was looking more and more bipolarish to me. Remember, she carried the legacy of sexual abuse and post-traumatic stress disorder—harbingers, in my mind at least, of bipolarity. I prescribed the mood-stabilizing Seroquel and gave her some samples to start with. The electricity feelings went away quickly on the drug, but when she had exhausted the free samples and tried to get her prescription filled, she found it prohibitively expensive.

"Anita, we haven't talked about this too much before, but I am wondering if you don't have bipolar disorder just like your daughter. It does run in families. We talked about mood shifts several years ago when you first came to me. Do you still have those?"

"Yes, but they are mostly with my period, and that is when I have my pain."

"Are you subject to mind-racing?"

"Oh am I! I have had that a long time—probably since I was a teenager."

"I am prescribing the drug, Lamictal. We will start at a low dose, and I want you to build it up gradually. Call me if you develop a rash, and I will see you back in three weeks."

Lamictal is about as expensive as Seroquel, but I had lots of samples to give her.

"It is the best drug yet. I can tell that my moods aren't swinging as much. I was not as uncomfortable with my last period, and my pain is really getting better."

"That's great. We are going to keep pushing the dose up slowly, and I will see you back in a month."

After five years of trying, I had finally found the right drug. If I had known more about the bipolar spectrum when I first saw her, it probably would not have taken nearly so long. Nonetheless, she was better, and I was content. It went well for about a year, and then on a routine visit I noticed that she was losing a little ground. She told me she was having more pain, and her mind was racing again. She was also getting more depressed. I offered to increase the dose of Lamictal. She thought it not necessary. It was a family matter, she told me, that was upsetting her. She really didn't want any change in her medicines, at least yet. At that juncture Anita was taking Klonopin, Lamictal, Neurontin, Nortriptyline, Hydrocodone, and Ritalin.

A few weeks later, I took a call from a psychiatry resident telling me that Anita had been admitted to the hospital for suicidal depression. We spoke at some length, and I told the doctor that I felt our patient had bipolar disorder and that, at least until now, the Lamictal had been a very helpful drug for her. The resident told me she concurred with my diagnosis and would certainly continue the Lamictal. She felt the Hydrocodone and Klonopin, however, well-known for their depressant effects, would have to be terminated. I commented that such drugs can be very helpful in the bipolar, particularly the bipolar in pain. Surprisingly, the resident said she had heard of that effect but felt that discontinuing the drugs was appropriate. I made no protestation. My patient had failed my care, so why not let someone else take over? But I sure didn't think Hydrocodone and Klonopin had caused her depression. She had been on them for five years and had found them helpful.

Good-bye, Anita. You are in the hands of others, and I hope you do well.

Somewhat to my surprise, she reappeared within a few weeks, and she looked quite well.

"I am doing better, Dr. Cochran. They had some counseling sessions when I was in the hospital that were very helpful. I can assure you I am not going to commit suicide. But I have to tell you, when they took my meds away from me, I started hurting badly, and I was having a lot of trouble sleeping. As soon as I got home I got back on them. I am still on the Lamictal, and I am feeling well now. Will you let me continue the medicines you had me on before?"

"Of course I will, but you must tell me what has been going on. I remember when I saw you last you were unwell. Something was troubling you. Something was making your bipolar disease come to the fore. What was it?"

"It wasn't the drugs, Dr. Cochran. It wasn't the drugs at all. It was my pregnant, unwed, teenage daughter that made me want to commit suicide. I have a new grandchild now, my first. It didn't happen the way I wanted it to happen, but I am going to love that child, and I am going to help take care of her."

"I'll write the drugs for you, Anita, and congratulations on your new grandchild. It just may be a restorative experience for you. Loving a new grandchild can do that to a woman."

"I am learning that."

"Anita, how long were you in the hospital?"

"Five days."

"What was it like? How did they treat you?"

"They treated me like a dog, like I was a drug addict, and I am not making that up! I overheard the nurses talking about me."

"I regret that. There was no reason for you to be treated that way."

"Well, I was, and I resolved that I was going to get well quick and get out of that place."

Everybody knows, or thinks they know, that drugs such as opiates and benzodiazepines can cause depression. I have learned since I have become a pain doctor that if everybody knows it, it is often wrong. In my experience, these drugs are more often antidepressant than depressant, and I have certainly demonstrated that in the stories of those in pain. It is convenient to *blame* the opiates for, as we shall see, just about anything that goes wrong. They are a handy culprit, and in the rest of this chapter, I will tell you of those whose illness was blamed inappropriately on opiates.

Rachael Morningstar was Cherokee. She had a high place in the Indian nation and was frequently a dancer at their gatherings. She suffered chronic back pain following an automobile accident and also fibromyalgia with pain throughout her body. She acknowledged sexual abuse in her youth at the hands of a half brother who, she said, was "sociopathic." She told me also that she suffered severe emotional abuse from a supervisor at work who "tortured me." This led to her termination from employment with city government. She suffered post-traumatic stress disorder and was chronically depressed. Some two years before coming me she attempted suicide. Following that she was diagnosed with bipolar disorder and treated with Cymbalta and Lamictal. She told me that her treatment notwithstanding, she remained depressed. She continued to have spells of sleeplessness and high energy when she would "bounce off the walls." I began treatment with Imipramine, Klonopin, and Hydrocodone to be taken every four hours as needed for pain.

Her response was at best partial, and I elected early on to add Ritalin. It can be uniquely beneficial in the bipolar, and moreover her depression had really not responded very well to any of the conventional antidepressants or mood stabilizers. She did well, at least for a while, until her father died of lung cancer. She crashed, and her sociopathic brother also. They argued incessantly, and he, she said, threatened to kill her. She obtained a restraining order against him saying he was "torturing me," the same words she had used to describe the supervisor who had so abused her. I suppose what she told me was the truth, but one wonders if there might not have been an element of paranoia.

As time went by she became ever more painful and also irritable and angry. I added Methadone. There were problems with nausea at first, but she came to tolerate the drug and was enthusiastic about it.

"It has helped my attitude as much as my pain. I feel human again."

She got a couple of good years out of her medications. And then another event—the death of her mother. With it came altercations with her brother and then suicidal despair and rage.

"I had to go back into the hospital, Dr. Cochran. I was there for two weeks."

"Tell me about it."

"My diagnosis was bipolar disorder and paranoia."

"Were you seeing or hearing things that weren't there?"

"How did you know that? I was hearing things, threatening things."

"Who was your doctor?"

"Well, I don't even remember the name of the first one, but he was the most arrogant man I have ever seen. He came into my room, and without introducing himself or asking about how I was feeling said, 'You are a drug addict.' That angered me, Dr. Cochran. It angered me a lot. I told him I wasn't a drug addict, that I was manic-depressive, suicidal, and hallucinating. I told him I needed more support than he was going to give me, and I refused to accept him as a doctor, so they sent me to another one, a Dr. Adewola."

"I know of him. He is highly regarded."

"He was really nice, and I liked him a lot. He was very gentle with me. He told me I wasn't a drug addict, but that the pain medicine and Ritalin might be contributing to my hallucinations. He told me he would have to taper them, and he started me on a medicine called Risperdal. My hallucinations and depression started getting better, but it did take a while. Like I told you, I was in there two weeks."

"That's a pretty long hospital stay in this day and age."

"Yes, it took that long. I have to tell you that off my pain medicine, I was hurting badly. I think I would have gotten better sooner if they kept me on the drugs. As soon as I left the hospital I got back on them. I started on a low dose and built it up over a week, and I am feeling a lot better now."

"Does Dr. Adewola know that you are back on the medicines?"

"Yes, I told him. I was very frank with him. He said it was just fine. He agreed that the opiates and Ritalin I was on probably had nothing to do with my illness. He even acknowledged that they might be helping my bipolar disorder."

"That's interesting."

I don't think I have ever had a patient taking opiates who was admitted to a psychiatric hospital and *not* withdrawn from the drugs. I do understand the conventional wisdom that opiates are bad for mental health, but I certainly don't agree with it.

There are times when it is mandatory to remove a person from opiates, and I have referenced this already. Cardiographic changes or cardiac or respiratory symptoms demand that the drugs be stopped. Otherwise, I am really not sure that we need to be so negatively knee-jerk reactive to opiates in the emotionally unwell.

If Rachael had not been removed from her opiate and stimulant therapy, would she indeed have gotten well quicker? I suspect so. They had supported her and maintained emotional equilibrium for years. It was only under the stress of her mother's death and threatening altercations with her half brother did she begin to hallucinate. We can't blame my therapy for that.

Gloria was about sixty when she came to me. She was many years under psychiatric care, taking the antidepressant, Effexor, which she told me controlled her mood like no other drug she had ever taken. Her major problem was chronic neck pain following several operations. I prescribed Hydrocodone, and she got good pain relief. It was necessary for me to see her only every six months for a quick check and prescription refills.

A few years into treatment, I took a phone call from her primary care physician. He was concerned about her opiate use. On a recent visit she appeared quite impaired to him. I thanked him for his call and told him I would bring her in for an evaluation.

I have learned, regrettably, that the belief that opiates always impair those who take them is epidemic in the medical community. So much so that I never accept the diagnosis of drug intoxication or impairment made by another physician, however esteemed that colleague may be. I reserve the right to judge myself if my patient is intoxicated or impaired from opiates.

I found nothing on my examination of Gloria to indicate there was a problem. Speech was fluent. Her gait was somewhat hesitant and slow but nothing of alarm. I tracked her prescription history and saw no indication of overuse of the drug. She told me it was continuing to help her, and I saw no reason at all to discard it.

Within a few weeks I received another call, this one much more confrontational.

"Dr. Cochran, you have got to get this woman off Hydrocodone. She came by for blood tests today, and my nurses told me that she was very impaired."

"Impaired in what way?"

"They told me she was slow and lethargic and that her speech was slurred. You really need to get her off that drug."

"Okay, I will take another look."

This time I saw what he was talking about. Gloria was *bradykinetic*, that is, there was a poverty of movement. Her gait was slower than I had seen before, and the swing of her arms while walking was diminished. Her speech, however, to my ear was normal. Bradykinesia is a hallmark of Parkinson's disease. I searched for other signs of the disorder but found neither tremor nor muscular rigidity.

Gloria told me she had an appointment to see a neurologist because she was aware that she was slowing down some, and she had another symptom, a very strange one. She felt cold all the time. She had to wear heavy clothes to protect her. None of her doctors, it seemed, had been able to figure out why she felt this way.

I couldn't explain it either, but I thought there was at least a possibility that my patient was in an early stage of Parkinson's. I wrote her a prescription for Sinemet, the usual start-up for the disorder, and I told her to be sure and take the prescription bottle to the neurologist she was about to see. Her response to the drug would be helpful information for him. Satisfied that I had performed my obligations, and satisfied that my patient was not drug-intoxicated, I scheduled a return for routine refills in six months.

She was worse, much worse. Her speech had changed. She was *dysarthric*. She sounded like she was talking with a mouthful of food. Her gait was even slower than before, and she exhibited a strange tremor of her tongue. It was periodically protruding through her lips sometimes at the corner of her mouth and sometimes from the center.

"Gloria, did you take the Sinemet that I prescribed?"

"Yes, it made me sick at my stomach, and the neurologist told me I didn't have Parkinson's disease anyway."

"What did he say you did have?"

"He didn't know, but he is going to do an MRI on my brain to see why I feel so cold all the time."

"Gloria, are you aware that your tongue is moving about? It keeps protruding between your lips."

"Yes, I have noticed that, and I can't control it. It came on after I got some new dentures. I guess that's what is causing it."

Her tremor was *orofacial dyskinesia*. It is a not uncommon tremor, and it is almost always produced by drug therapy, most commonly by the antipsychotics. Gloria was taking no such drug, but she had been taking Effexor for many years from her psychiatrist. I looked the drug up in the *Physician's Desk Reference*, and sure enough, there it was. Bradykinesia and orofacial dyskinesia, also known as *tardive dyskinesia* (because it appears late, after years of the use of a drug) can occasionally occur with Effexor.

Her psychiatrist accepted my call, and I told him of my observations. He recognized that dyskinesia could occur with the Effexor therapy. He told me he would see her promptly. I hope it plays out well, but it may not. Sometimes the dyskinesia gets worse when the offending drug is stopped. I hope that is not the case with Gloria. And I wonder about her unnatural feeling of coldness. Could that possibly be a drug effect also? I suspect so.

Now back to the doctor who called me in such a confrontational manner telling me I must remove our mutual patient from her Hydrocodone therapy. Was he so blinded by the belief that opiates impair that he failed to recognize that other drugs also impair? Effexor was the culprit, not the opiate. Gloria had a disease that should have been recognized sooner had not his focus, and therefore mine, been so directed to her opiate usage.

Ethel was introduced to me by a fax from her primary care physician. She was seventy-five years old and chronically in pain from advanced and widespread arthritis. Her doctor had prescribed Hydrocodone, but with the passage of time, Ethel began exhibiting unusual behaviors that strongly suggested drug abuse to him. My counsel was requested.

Ethel told me that Hydrocodone was helping her and that she was taking it as prescribed. She acknowledged severe depression since the death of her husband five years before. Also, since his death, difficulty with her daughter, whom she said was "controlling." My evaluation completed, I concluded that my new patient was severely depressed and also in a very dysfunctional relationship with her only child. I reviewed the Board of Pharmacy Web site that allows me to obtain a medication history, and I saw no evidence of overuse of the prescribed drug. I maintained her Hydrocodone and added Zoloft. I suggested that counseling for both Ethel and her daughter might be very helpful. It seemed to me that their relationship was a major, if not the major problem, in this woman's illness.

Ethel scoffed at the idea saying, "That will never happen. She is just too controlling to submit to something like that. You see, I'm the problem, not her."

I saw Ethel for several months, and I made little headway at all. Her pain was being controlled fairly well with the Hydrocodone, but the reader is advised that no pain drug works very well in the face of a severe depression. I tried several different antidepressants but none worked. Then another fax from the referring doctor. Ethel was clearly drug-intoxicated. Her daughter had been in communication with him several times and was extremely concerned. I called and acknowledged receipt of the fax and suggested that Ethel and her daughter come in together for my evaluation. I was told that the daughter was more than prepared to do that. An appointment was made.

When I entered the exam room, Ethel was in a wheelchair, her back to me. She was facing her daughter, so it was the daughter's countenance that I first saw when I entered. She was an attractive woman. I would put her age about forty-five. She was wearing a very handsome pale blue suit, unusually formal attire for a visit to the doctor, I thought. Her emotional bearing was, shall I use the word, focused. It was not an unpleasant visage, but it wasn't especially pleasant either. Moreover, she was holding a camcorder in her lap. I knew I was confronting a woman on a mission.

I seated myself and then turned to Ethel. I asked how she was doing, and she gave me a big smile and then extended her arm and hand to me as if requesting a high five. I gave her one, and then she said, "Hiya, buddy." That greeting completed, she extended her knees up toward the ceiling with her skirt dropping to show more thigh than I wanted to see.

"Whoops," she said.

Oh boy, I thought, this is going to take some processing!

"Dr. Cochran, we have to get Mother off the Hydrocodone. It is making her act really strangely. Here, please look at the camcorder. I want you to see what is going on."

"Forgive me, but not yet. I need to go over this chart and review all that has happened."

"Very well."

Ethel gave me another high five and again said, "Hiya, buddy." I reviewed as quickly as I could all that had transpired and been recorded in my medical records. The original fax from her doctor telling me that she was impaired and probably abusing her drugs, then my evaluation that our core problem here was unremitting depression and, since the death of her husband, conflict with her daughter. Months of unsuccessful treatment for depression. Then the second fax imploring me to take action, and that is where we stood at that juncture. I directed my attention and conversation to the daughter because Ethel was babbling away nonsensically.

"I have always thought the major problem here was depression since the death of her husband a few years ago. Is that correct?"

"Oh, Dr. Cochran, she has been depressed all her life. Mother does have her idiosyncrasies. Every now and then she would act a little bit bizarre but nothing like this."

The daughter was becoming a bit more engaging and a little less stern in appearance. Perhaps she had sized me up and decided I was not the drug-pushing ogre she expected me to be.

"Has she ever seen a psychiatrist?"

"No."

"You say she has been acting strangely, and I can certainly see that. How long has it been this bad?"

"Off and on since she has been on the pain medicine, but it is getting a lot worse. I am sure the Hydrocodone is the problem."

"When was she started on the pain medicine?"

"When my father died. Dr. Cochran, I really want you to look at this camcorder. You will be astonished."

"I really don't need to. I have seen enough."

And I had. In a span of but a few minutes I had made a diagnosis, and it wasn't drug intoxication. Unlike those so afflicted, Ethel's speech, although largely nonsensical, was quite fluent. There was no slurring of her words. Her motor skills were intact. Her high fives and knee-lifts were performed from a wheelchair with acrobatic proficiency. What I was seeing was not intoxication. It was disinhibition.

"Daughter, this behavior is not due to the drug. This is bipolar mania. That is what you are looking at."

There was several seconds of hesitation while she absorbed what I had told her. I have to give her a lot of credit. There was no denial. There was no anger. When recognition finally came, her tears began to flow. She said

"Oh my God!" She then fell to her knees and embraced her mother who was still talking rapidly and nonsensically.

"What can we do, Dr. Cochran? We have to do something."

"She needs psychiatric hospitalization, and I can't do that. I am not a psychiatrist, but you can take her to the hospital. I will arrange for a social worker to do an intake interview. The gold standard for psychiatric admission in this day is whether the patient is a danger to themselves or others, and your mother clearly is. I am sure they will admit her and place her under the care of competent psychiatrist."

I made the necessary phone call and introduced the patient who would appear at the hospital shortly. I was called back a couple of hours later and told that she was indeed manic and was being admitted.

Poor Ethel. Her daughter and her doctor had been barking up the wrong tree for several years. Idiosyncrasies and occasional bizarre behaviors were probably expressions of mania, and there is no doubt that what I had witnessed was. Recall the daughter telling me that mother "has been depressed all her life." Why did it take so many years to finally come to a correct diagnosis? And why was it so easy to blame her abnormal behaviors on her opiate therapy?

In this chapter, we have seen opiates blamed for suicide threats, for paranoia and hallucinations, for tardive dyskinesia, and now for mania. In no case at all were they in any way operative. I am afraid that we physicians often wear diagnostic blinders when we attend those who take opiates regularly.

"Bob, I want to refer a patient to you, and I need to apologize because I have found her very unpleasant and difficult to deal with. I am treating her for breast cancer, and we are concluding her chemotherapy now. One of my problems is that she is always requesting pain medicine for her headache. I refused to give her any. I told her that I was an oncologist, and it was my responsibility to treat her cancer, not her headaches. But she continues to be very insistent that I give her something for pain. I've learned that she has been getting Hydrocodone from several different doctors. She is obviously drug-seeking and probably abusing. She went to the emergency room last night drug intoxicated. Again, I hate to ask you to see her, but sometimes you do pretty well with people like this."

"Well, I will give it a try. Please send me some of her medical records—that will help a lot."

I was stunned when I first saw Molly. It wasn't her chemo-induced baldness. It was her youth. She was thirty years old, she told me, and her mastectomy had been performed a year before. Breast cancer at age twenty-nine! Maybe the oncologist was used to seeing such things, but I wasn't. It touched me deeply, and I found myself liking my new patient a lot.

I continued my inquiries. She told me that she was eight years into a very good marriage with two children. She described a traumatic childhood with an alcoholic father but denied physical or sexual abuse. She told me that "my childhood made me stronger." She had never been troubled with anxiety or depression until she was diagnosed with breast cancer and begun on treatment with Effexor. Migraines first appeared at her age eighteen, and she went under the care of a neurologist taking drugs such as Lamictal and Amitriptyline. Perhaps they worked, but it is hard to be sure because after three or four years, her migraines abated to be replaced with an incessant viselike generalized headache. She was told she had analgesic rebound headaches and advised to stop all pain medicines, even over-the-counter drugs, which she did totally without benefit. (She didn't have analgesic rebound headaches. She had transformed migraine. Why it should develop when she was young, happily married, and bearing children, I don't know.)

Along the way she was given Hydrocodone, but she told me she never took it regularly, and she certainly never abused it. However, since the breast cancer, her headaches had become more intense, and her primary care doctor, she lied, was giving her Hydrocodone on a regular basis.

I continued my explorations and learned that throughout her life she had been subject to very vivid dreams. She awoke from them neither emotional nor paralyzed but with the sensation that her whole body was on fire. That would last ten minutes or so. She did acknowledge some daytime sleepiness.

"Molly, I spoke with your oncologist, and she told me that you had to go to the emergency room a few days ago. Could you tell me about that?"

"I'll tell you as much as I can remember, but a lot of it I don't remember. I was at a dentist office awaiting an appointment, and I started feeling strange, just not right. I don't know how to describe it. And then I had a sense of numbness and tingling in the right side of my face and my hand. I stood up and wobbled to the receptionist and tried to tell her that something was happening to me and that I needed help, but I couldn't speak. I couldn't make a sound. The receptionist called my husband, and he came and took me to the emergency room. By that time I was really confused, and I don't remember much of the rest—only that after I left the emergency room and my husband was driving me home, I had an intense headache. It was the worst migraine I have ever endured. It lasted several hours, and then I was able to go to sleep. When I woke up the next day the headache and numbness were gone, and I could speak normally. My husband told me that the doctors in the emergency room said I was drug-intoxicated from Hydrocodone."

It didn't take me long to process what she told me. One does not suddenly become drug-intoxicated waiting for a dental appointment. That exercise, as we have seen, can be anxiety-producing, and the appearance of migraine while one is awaiting a dental appointment requires no stretch of the imagination.

Many migraineurs experience an *aura* at the onset of the attack. It is usually characterized by nausea, a change in mood, and visual effects such as scintillations. This is known in current parlance as *migraine with aura*. However, the aura can be much more complex and can be attended by confusion, numbness in the face and extremities, and arrest of speech. This, in medical parlance, is known as *complicated migraine*, and it should never have been misdiagnosed as drug intoxication. But it was. It is so easy to blame opiates for any alteration of behavior. They are such a convenient culprit.

I elected to prescribe Klonopin and Ritalin for she certainly had features of narcolepsy, albeit atypical, and she certainly had chronic pain. I gave her Hydrocodone also at her requested dose of 10 mg three times daily.

Before I began dictating my consultation note to the oncologist, I took a quick look at the medical records that had been forwarded to me. They were most interesting.

> "Molly returns today for a third cycle of Taxotere and Cytoxin. We have had a number of issues with her over the past several weeks. We learned that she had taken at least 90 Hydrocodone over the past two months. These had come from several doctors. She recently sustained a fall and a superficial laceration over her right eye. She was diagnosed with strep throat and given Amoxicillin and a Hydrocodone cough syrup. She took it over a 24 hour time period and developed slurred speech. Her family took her car keys away at my recommendation, and her speech improved.

I confronted her about the amount of medication she was taking including narcotics. She tells me she has a significant problem with headaches and migraines. She has been placed on several medications, and none of these have helped her headaches at all over the past years. She is agitated and distraught over my confrontation. She is crying and yelling and threatening to leave as well as to not complete her chemotherapy. Her mother is here and confirms her aberrant behavior as well as volatile emotions but has not noticed that her daughter has a drug addiction problem."

Slurred speech while on Hydrocodone cough syrup on top of Hydrocodone taken for pain. What did that mean? Probably a transient intoxication due to accidental overdosage. I should have paid more attention to her mother's acknowledgement of "aberrant behavior as well as volatile emotions." Instead, I elected to explore Molly's drug usage. I went to the Board of Pharmacy Web site. She was indeed receiving Hydrocodone from several doctors and from several different drug stores—a clear sign of manipulation and abuse. However, I have learned to view all things related to pain and all things drug-abusing with a jaundiced eye. Thankfully so, because I realized that Molly's use of Hydrocodone from multiple doctors amounted to ninety 10-mg pills a month. It is by no means an excessive dose, and it was exactly the amount she requested from me. I saw that each of her three doctors was providing her with thirty Hydrocodone pills a month. I wondered if Molly was going to three doctors because no one of them would prescribe a quantity sufficient to control her pain. Maybe she was not abusing drugs after all, and maybe her lie that she was getting her drugs from her primary care doctor was to protect herself from the prejudice that befalls those who get pain medicines from multiple doctors.

On her return, she told me she was much better. Her headaches had diminished in severity, and she was no longer suffering fearful dreams and awakening from them with intense pain. I was pleased with her progress, and I told her to continue the same medications, and that I would see her again in a month. I received a letter before her next appointment. It was from her oncologist.

Dear Bob:

Thank you very much for seeing Molly Henderson.
I know that a thank-you note may not be adequate, but
I believe you have really helped her significantly. Her
headaches are so much better that she is able to have a more
normal quality of life, and this has made all the difference
for her.

Thank you again for what you are doing.

Sincerely,
Betty Ralston, MD

A nice letter of appreciation, but perhaps also a letter of contrition, for
Dr. Ralston had deemed our patient as unpleasant and drug-abusing.

Molly completed her chemotherapy, and her hair started coming back.
She continued to do well, and I enjoyed her visits because she was a very
engaging young woman. I thought I had a cure, but there were problems yet.

She had to be started on the drug, Tamoxifen. It is an estrogen
inhibitor, and its side effects can be daunting. Molly discovered that the
Tamoxifen caused her migraines to recur. Even if she broke the pill in half
and took it twice a day instead of the prescribed one, she would have a
migraine. Moreover, with Tamoxifen, her dreams were recurring, and she
was becoming depressed.

I increased the dose of Ritalin, and she did quite well, better than I
expected. She was able to continue the Tamoxifen, and although each half
pill gave her a slight headache, it was quite tolerable. I was pleased with
what had been achieved. Migraine, then transformed migraine, then breast
cancer, then depression, and then something approach a cure with Ritalin,
Klonopin, Effexor, and Hydrocodone. All was well, and I was at peace and
I thought Molly also.

Then calls from pharmacists telling me that she was requesting early
refills on the Hydrocodone. I learned she was getting her prescriptions
refilled every two weeks. She was taking 180 Hydrocodone a month, six
daily—far more than I prescribed. I called her in and confronted her, and
I will admit if I had been wiser and more patient, I could have done it
better. She became angry and agitated. She began to cry, and she entered
denial, telling me that she had never taken the medicines other than as I
had prescribed. I told her that I had evidence to the contrary. She grew ever
more angry, shouting at me.

"I have done nothing wrong. Those records you have are wrong. I have never done anything like what you say. You are accusing me. That is what you are doing. You are accusing me. I have never done anything wrong."

She was screaming, and she was angry and out of control. I should have realized that what I was seeing was the clinical equivalent of road rage. I wish I had recognized that before I initiated conversation again, and I wish I had recalled that the oncologist had confronted this same kind of angry behavior.

"Molly, you must understand I will have to discharge you from my care. You are not taking the Hydrocodone as I prescribed it. If you needed more, you should have told me. The dosage you are taking is actually within appropriate limits, but I can't provide it for you if you are going to lie to me. This is the end of our relationship, but I have to tell you, I don't think you are a bad person. But you are a person I have been unable to cure. Maybe your next doctor can do it. I couldn't, but I want you to know that I would like to help you. When you go to your new doctor, whoever he or she is, you can give them my name, and I will speak to them to support you."

She left angry and tearful.

I assure you, encounters such I have described are quite as painful to me as they are to the other party. I always wonder if I could have used more tact and employed more patience, but sometimes that is hard to do in the company of deceit. Her chart still in my hand, I went back to the oncologist's notes and read about the same kind of event I had experienced and also the words that "Her mother is here and confirms her aberrant behavior as well as volatile emotions."

I had not served my patient well. I had recognized her bipolar spectrum in the form of narcolepsy, migraines, and chronic headaches, and I had treated it rather well. I had failed, however, to address the issue of mood swings and rage. I should have, and she should have been more candid with me about her emotions and her drug usage. Was Molly using the Hydrocodone to control her moods? I'll never know, but I suspect it just might be something like that.

It was a couple of weeks later that I received a phone call from a neurologist at a pain clinic. She was inquiring about my experience with Molly. I recounted her history and told the doctor that Molly had been deceitful with me, taking much more of her drugs than I had prescribed, but that I did not think she was truly an addict. I suspected that her overuse was probably an attempt to treat not just her pain but her bipolar disorder also.

"Thank you so much for telling me all this. It helps me understand. I promise you, I will take good care of your patient. I will do everything I can to help her."

I do hope it turns out well for Molly. I hope she is more candid with the new doctor than with the old ones, and I hope the new doctor realizes that the next complicated migraine is just that and not opiate intoxication.

CHAPTER 15

Concluding

The discovery, or better, the rediscovery of the opiate cure, and I am by no means the only person to have done it, is, I believe, a clinical event of the first magnitude. The cures can be so dramatic, so sudden and total, that denial simply cannot be sustained. A clinical effect that but five years ago was said to be impossible is beginning to be recognized as at least possible if not probable.

What is the immediate *practical* use of the discovery? I believe it begins with pain doctors, those who are knowledgeable in opiate therapy and willing to prescribe the drugs. When they become more cognizant of the bipolar spectrum and all its ramifications, and some of them are doing so, they will, I hope, be more aggressive with their therapy and more aware that they may not only relieve pain but also bipolarity. When will other physicians who treat bipolar disorder, and I am referring to psychiatrists and primary care physicians, begin to employ opiates? It may take a while because of their lack of experience with opiate therapy and perhaps their fear, warranted or not, of the risk of addiction. Nonetheless, I think it is beginning to happen.

A young bipolar patient of mine with chronic pain stabilized immediately on Methadone. She did very well for a matter of a year or so and then, because of insurance issues, left my care. Unable to find another doctor who would prescribe the drug, she entered suicidal despair and required three hospitalizations over the course of but a few months. The third time around, her psychiatrist finally accepted her declaration that Methadone and only Methadone controlled her moods. He administered it in the requested dose, 30 mg every eight hours, during her hospital stay and was able to witness her recovery. He told her at the time of her discharge from the hospital that he was unable to provide ongoing opiate therapy for her. He suggested that she return to me for she now had Medicare coverage and insurance resources. I applaud his effort. I am sure that was the first time in the history of that psychiatric hospital that an opiate had been administered to control mental illness. It was done, however, in a highly controlled environment where nurses could witness her behavior and provide the drug in the appropriate quantity at the appropriate interval. That control would not be available when she went home, and I am sure the psychiatrist was fearful of drug misuse. Still, he had witnessed the opiate cure cure, and he won't forget it.

Another promising note. A psychiatrist sent me a referral letter that was most interesting. He had been struggling with an unstable bipolar, refractory to all the medicines he had prescribed. She faced electroconvulsive therapy as a last resort, and he thought, as he charmingly wrote, "Your way of thinking just might help her." I can't wait to see her.

Let's revisit the first chapter of this book in which I listed the various drugs useful for the treatment of bipolar disorder. The anxiolytics can be quite helpful although their usage is disdained by some who view their risk of addiction, sedation, and loss of balance as a threat to their long-term employ. The tricyclic and tricyclic-like antidepressants carry the risk of sedation and also faints due to low blood pressure. They also cause weight gain. The SSRIs can be weight-gaining and also sex-inhibiting. They do carry a risk of suicidal ideation and attempt, and we are increasingly recognizing the side effect of intestinal hemorrhage. The mood stabilizing anticonvulsants carry the risk collectively of sedation and in some of them, weight gain, liver damage, skin rash, or reduced white blood cell count. The older antipsychotics, of which Thorazine is an example, produce tremors, and I have already exampled dyskinesia and akathisia. Unlike many side effects, these particular ones do not necessarily go away when the drug is discontinued. The newer antipsychotics carry a diminished risk of tremor, but in its place we have the very real risk of obesity and particularly the induction of diabetes.

Be aware that all of these drugs are used over the long term because bipolar disorder is a long-term disease. And the longer the usage, the greater the risk of side effects. You have certainly realized from this text (and perhaps from your own experience) that none of these drugs are a panacea. They often don't work, and sometimes they work for a while and then stop working. They are, all of them, a long way from perfect.

Now where does opiate therapy fit with the benefit/risk ratio? Perhaps surprisingly to you, long-term opiate therapy has rather few side effects. It can be sedating but so can most of the conventional psychopharmaceuticals. Importantly, the opiates only rarely cause weight gain, and they almost never cause tremors (indeed, they relieve tremors). I am unaware of a particularly high incidence of suicide attempt on opiate therapy and certainly no problem with intestinal bleeding. I do have to acknowledge a very important side effect of opiate therapy, and that is an increased incidence of sudden, presumably cardiac, deaths. The incidence, it seems, is greatest with Methadone. The problem has attracted great attention. It does appear the cardiac problems with Methadone can be predicted by changes in the electrocardiogram, and routine monitoring is now standard operating procedure. Be advised that Methadone is not the only drug that produces cardiac arrhythmias. There are dozens of nonopiate drugs, including some antidepressants, that carry the same threat.

It took me forty-five years as a physician to overcome my ignorance and my bias and to realize that opiates are among the safest drugs we have. They do carry the risk of addiction, but, as I have emphasized, the incidence is really rather low. When the drugs do what they are supposed to do, control pain and the many symptoms of the bipolar spectrum, addiction is quite uncommon. And only rarely have I seen the equivalent of the sudden and total recovery that is the opiate cure equaled by conventional psychopharmacy.

Now let's look at the benefit/risk analysis of the other competitor to the opiate cure, and that is electroconvulsive therapy. It is the gold standard for the treatment of depression, and that includes bipolar depression. It is reserved for those who do not respond to pharmacotherapy, and there is no question it can be extremely helpful. It doesn't always work, though, and although its application is more refined than formerly, it still carries the significant risk of permanent memory impairment, and that, I assure you, is quite a severe side effect.

So where does opiate therapy in the bipolar stand in relation to pharmacotherapy or electroconvulsive therapy? I believe that if the bipolar patient has chronic pain in any of its various expressions, the institution of opiate and/or stimulant therapy can be undertaken after but a brief trial of more conventional therapy. The rewards are just too great to be ignored. Now how about the bipolar *without* a pain problem? And realize that we really don't know yet whether the opiates will work as well in the bipolar who is not in pain as they do in the one that is in pain. We may be dealing with two different diseases, but that seems rather unlikely. I would propose opiate therapy only after failure or intolerance to multiple more conventional drugs. I would, however, advocate a therapeutic trial of opiates and/or stimulants before submitting a person to therapeutic electroconvulsion. As an aside, I have several patients who have failed electroconvulsive therapy but who responded to opiates or stimulants. Why not try them first?

The opiate cure offers an enormous *conceptual* advance. Its discovery, almost simultaneously with the recognition of the bipolar spectrum, will, I believe, change many of our current views about mental illness. It will change our custom of recognizing several different individual psychiatric disorders as distinct and separate entities. They are not. Their overlap, one with another, both clinically and therapeutically, is, if the case studies I have offered have any credibility, irrefutable. At the risk of repetition, recall that I have, with opiate therapy, relieved mood-shifting bipolarity, narcolepsy, attention deficiency, obsessive-compulsive disorder, post-traumatic stress disorder, and multiple personality disorder. I have also relieved a variety of symptoms including pain, tremors such as akathisia and Tourette's, compulsive hair-pulling, obsessive worry, nocturia, even salt and opiate cravings, and for heaven's sake, self-mutilation! I have offered the case histories of many people who suffered several of these disorders simultaneously who have experienced relief of all by the administration of a class of drugs whose parent, the opium poppy, has been used medicinally as best we can tell from historical records, for some six thousand years. It staggers my imagination, and my imagination is not easily staggered.

I have already suggested that all of these diseases and symptoms may actually be the product of some lack or inefficiency in the brain's opioid systems. If that is indeed true, and the case studies in this book suggest that it certainly might be, it will mandate that we appropriately prescribe opiates for the treatment of mental illness. It will also mandate the creation of a new science, that of opiate psychopharmacology, the study of just why and how and in whom these drugs work so well for so many different disorders.

Lastly, let's address the opiate cure as a *societal* issue. My wife of over fifty years had progressive spinal deterioration and required a six-hour operation, a fusion, to correct her deformity. Her orthopedist prescribed, quite appropriately, Oxycodone for relief of her postoperative pain, and she did well on only 10 mg twice daily. She is several years removed from her surgery, and her care has fallen to her internist, and he has, without hesitation, continued that therapy. He is a wise man, and he has no particular concern at all over the ongoing use of the drug. He does not feel, as some physicians certainly do, that she should be taken *off* opiate therapy simply because she is *on* it. Perhaps she could get by without the drug, but why bother? She is doing well, and if it ain't broke, don't fix it.

She takes sixty 10 mg pills a month, and our cost under Medicare D prescription drug plan is three dollars. The value of the Oxycodone (and most other opiates) on the street is a dollar per milligram. Thus, the sale of her Oxycodone, if we chose to do so, would bring in six hundred dollaes a month—an enormous profit on investment.

The abuse and diversion of opiates begins with the obscene profit generated by their illicit sales. There are many links in our society's drug abuse issue, and I will discuss them, but remember always, it begins with profit. I am sure that some of my patients, given drugs that I prescribe appropriately, choose to sell them to others. This happens to me and every other doctor who prescribes opiates. I try to control my practice quite carefully, and I think the number of people who sell drugs prescribed by me is rather low. A much more common problem is theft of drugs for resale from people who were legitimately prescribed them. In this book I have given you an example of theft of opiates by family members. I remember well an elderly bipolar whose pharmacist alerted me to the fact that she was getting early fills on her prescriptions. She was wheelchair-bound, incapable of driving an automobile, and therefore someone else had to be picking up her medicines. When I confronted her, she admitted that she had known all along that her granddaughter was getting her prescriptions filled and selling them to buy new clothes. My patient told me she had endured great pain in the absence of her opiates, but she did not want to confront or prosecute her granddaughter. When it all finally came to light, the child was denied entry into her grandmother's home. The problem was resolved but hardly satisfactorily.

It is remarkable to me just how carelessly many of my patients handle their drugs. They misplace and lose them. They leave them in insecure places in their automobiles and in their homes where family, guests, or house cleaners come. It is no coincidence that the reported theft of drugs increases during holiday seasons when people open their homes to guests, some of whom they really don't know very well. I am sure some of my patients are lying to me when they tell me their drugs have been stolen, but I believe most of the time that they are telling me the truth. Theft of prescription drugs is rampant because the quest for easy profit is a temptation that many can't turn down.

I recently attended to a forty-five-year-old woman, an artisan, who was in great demand for her quilts. She was in the company of her husband, a rather large and plainly dressed man but one who exuded a certain sense of authority. I made my usual inquiries about her fibromyalgia and the many symptoms that so often accompany it. She was pretty much a closed book, and I really couldn't find many leads or clues, so I used a ploy. I asked if she had researched me, that is, gone to my Web site or read my books. As I have written many times in this book, patients are more forthcoming when they know more about me and the way I think. My patient responded that she had not, that she simply trusted her referring doctor and, therefore, made no effort to find out more about me.

Then her husband said, "I sure have researched you."

"Good, what do you think about what I do?"

He stood up, extended his hand to shake mine, and said, "You are okay, you are legitimate." He then gave me his card. He was a captain in the police department in a southern city in charge of the division investigating prescription drug fraud and abuse.

"You know, Dr. Cochran, there are lots of pain clinics out there, and some of them are pretty bad."

"I am somewhat aware of that."

"They see their patients every month. They charge three hundred dollars for the visit, and they give the patient anything they want."

"And they don't accept insurance, do they?"

"Absolutely not."

The profit motive again. There is enormous profit to be made by dispensing drugs legally, if hardly legitimately.

Now let's change gears a bit. "They give them anything they want." Or could they be giving them anything they *need*?

Just who are these people who are paying outrageous prices either to drug dealers or to doctors? Are they all addicts? I suppose some are, but I am quite sure that some are not. They are people with chronic pain and often bipolar disease who will pay any price for the control of their illness, and they do so because they are unable to gain control with the drugs and the dosages that their physicians prescribe. I have given you examples throughout this book of people who have illegally shared, purchased, or perhaps even stolen the drugs that relieve their emotional and physical discomfort. You must realize, if this book is any indicator, that we have drugs, the opiates that, it seems, can cure almost anything. They are indeed panaceas. No wonder people will pay outrageous prices for a cure. How many "drug abusers" are trying to control their bipolar disease and all of its manifestations? How many are taking drugs for the relief of their post-traumatic stress disorder? And how many for other diseases and other symptoms?

I have a local and regional reputation as a physician, hopefully as a knowledgeable one, who is willing to prescribe opiates in the appropriate circumstances, sometimes in high doses. Not a few people request my consultation and tell me that they regularly purchase medicines off the street for control of their pain or emotional state. All of them, almost without exception, deplore the fact that they must do this for control of their symptoms, for the ability to keep a job and raise a family. They are ashamed of their behavior, but they tell me there is no recourse. After exercising due diligence and satisfying myself that the person has a disorder, usually bipolarity, who is amenable to opiate therapy, I will prescribe the appropriate drug; and in my experience, addictive behavior almost never occurs.

Now let's look at another link in the drug abuse issue, and it is the physician. If the person using drugs, illicitly obtained, is relieved of his physical or mental illness, why does he not report it to his physician and request his prescription legally, legitimately, and, therefore, more cheaply?

Don't make me laugh.

You know the answer. It is not just because the physician doesn't know of the opiate cure. Even if he did, he would probably be fearful of prescribing opiates to one who volunteered that he bought them off the street and was therefore an "addict." The opiate cure is real but also, unfortunately, is the opiate stigma.

What would happen if the physician, upon reviewing his patient's medical history, became convinced that the patient would indeed find relief from pain, depression, mood shifts, or flashbacks and therefore was willing to prescribe opiates? In doing so, he would solve several problems. He would relieve his patient's distress, always the prime motivator, and he would remove a "drug abuser" off the street. And the illegal dealer and the illegitimate physician would make one less obscene profit.

Could we physicians actually reduce opiate abuse by prescribing the drugs appropriately and—this is important—therefore generously? Could we reduce opiate abuse by prescribing more drugs? It is paradoxical, counterintuitive, and perhaps even dangerous; but it is worthy of thought. It is not going to happen soon, and I think the core reason is the distrust that exists between the physician and the person with chronic pain. We don't trust them, and that is why we have them sign drug contracts and why we do urine drug screens and pill counts. It is why we dispense the drugs not to the level of the *their* comfort but to the level of *our* comfort. This is the reason, I believe strongly, that so many people obtain medicines from multiple doctors and buy them off the street. People with chronic pain do not trust their doctors. This is why they lie and exercise deceit. They have to. We make them do it because we view them as drug seekers.

The opiate cure is out there. That was the easy part. The opiate stigma is out there too. That is going to be the hard part.

INDEX

P

R

Edwards Brothers Malloy
Thorofare, NJ USA
February 27, 2014